Clinical Applications

of

Herbal Medicine

Clinical Applications
of
Herbal Medicine

by

Dr. Paul Barney

Woodland Publishing, Inc.
Pleasant Grove, UT

About the Author

Dr. Paul Barney completed a Bachelor's of Science degree in Zoology at Brigham Young University and received his medical degree from the University of Utah. Since completing his internship residency in family practice in 1982, Dr. Barney has been in private practice doing primary care family practice and emergency room medicine. He is also an adjunct professor at Weber State University and has lectured extensively on natural medicines.

In an effort to offer additional treatments to his patients, especially for conditions that do not respond well to traditional methods, Dr. Barney became interested in acupuncture and subsequently completed the acupuncture training course at the University of California at Los Angeles and is currently a member of the American Academy of Medical Acupuncture. His training in acupuncture led him to explore Chinese Herbal medicine, but the difficulty in accessing Chinese herbs created the incentive to learn more about Western herbal medicine. Dr. Barney has been using herbs in his practice for over five years.

Dedication

To my wife Deb, and our children Spencer, Chad, Siri, Seth, Cami, Shelli and Clint—some of my reasons to remain healthy.

Table of Contents

INTRODUCTION

THE MODERN DOCTOR AND ALTERNATIVE MEDICINE

I find it interesting that alternative medicine has experienced a tremendous growth in popularity in America in the past 25 years and that medical doctors, for the most part, have not been very involved. However, medical doctors may be partly responsible for this renewed interest in alternatives since many people are discovering that alternative therapies may be better for their particular conditions (with little or no side effects) and at a more reasonable cost when compared to treatments, surgeries, and prescription or over-the-counter medications prescribed by the doctor.

There seems to be a small group of doctors on one end of the spectrum who are opposed to most anything except conventional therapies. Then, there is a large group of doctors in the middle who tolerate or ignore their patients' use of alternative therapies. However, on the other end of the spectrum is a rapidly growing group of doctors who have developed a genuine interest in alternative therapies. I believe this last group represents the doctor of the future and, perhaps within the next decade we will see most doctors incorporating in their practices at least some therapies that today are considered alternatives.

There may be several reasons why more doctors are investigating alternative therapies today. In my case, I found that some patients and conditions did not respond well to the usual methods in which I had been trained. So, in an effort to help these people, I began investigating alternative therapies. Some doctors may explore alternative therapies in an attempt to better understand why their patients use them. Other doctors may explore alternative therapies in an effort to follow current trends.

So, why don't all doctors explore alternative therapies? Except for the small group of doctors opposed to alternatives, I believe most other doctors would integrate alternative therapies into their practices if it were not for two things. First, doctors spend eight or more years in school and time each week to keep up on the information within their particular specialty. The thought of spending another year or two learning about alternatives is often not very appealing. Second, even if a doctor decided to explore alternatives, where does he or she begin and where can a doctor find reliable information? Since almost all medical schools provide no education or

information on alternative therapies, proper sources becomes a big issu
However, the information exists and the doctors with a strong desire wi
persist in finding it—to the benefit of their patients.

THE MODERN PATIENT AND ALTERNATIVE MEDICINE

The patient is the real beneficiary of doctors investigating alternativ
medicine. Among the many alternative therapies, patients may find mor
effective methods for treating various diseases. Just as doctors adopt ne
ideas and methods, patients must be equally open to adjusting their way o
thinking since some alternative therapies, such as acupuncture, may be qui
unlike more familiar conventional therapies. Most objections by patients t
a new therapy are quickly overcome as they increase their understanding.
find it very helpful when patients are willing to open a book or as
questions so they better understand a new therapy.

Often, people who have little knowledge of herbs are concerned wit
the number of pills they are required to take every day when using herb
formulas. This is because we have become conditioned to the dosing o
modern, highly concentrated, single chemical component prescriptio
medications. Prescription drugs are often dosed at one to three pills a da
Those same active ingredients are found in herbs but in a less concentrate
form. I believe, as others who use a lot of herbal medicine, that there a
often many synergistic components within the herb that make the activ
ingredient more accessible to the body and more effective in lower dose
However, because of the lower concentration of actives in the herbs, it
often necessary to consume one pill three times a day and up to three o
four pills three times a day. As a point of interest, the Chinese doctor wi
often prescribe the equivalent of 100 or more pills a day in the form of
very concentrated tea. In general, even though this appears to be far beyon
what you would expect if you were taking a prescription medication, th
side effects are very infrequent when compared to many prescriptio
medications.

The belief if a little is good, a lot is better can be very dangerous wit
respect to both conventional and herbal medications. Occasionally, you w
find herbal preparations that are extremely concentrated, such as som
sophisticated European extracts, and are much like today's poten
prescription medicines. If you are not sure about a particular medicatio
don't guess. Wisdom and prudence should be used with all medicin
whether or not they are in a concentrated form. Also, unless otherwi

noted, it is best not to use herbs if you are pregnant or lactating without first consulting a health care professional who has good information on the subject.

Some patients may not find the help they are looking for from alternative therapies. And, as a doctor, I don't rely strictly on alternative therapies. If I feel a patient would be better off with a conventional therapy, that is what I recommend. Sometimes I feel a patient would be better off if they used both conventional and alternative therapies. In some cases, the conventional therapy is best and in some cases alternative methods are superior.

HERBAL FORMULAS

There are many different philosophies on how to best combine herbs into a formula. I have found a philosophy with which I feel very comfortable. Every formula I recommend in this book will have herbs that satisfy each of the following categories:

> active herbs (usually bitter)
> aromatic and carminative herbs
> demulcent herbs
> cleansing herbs

The idea behind this pattern is very simple. The active herbs provide the direct therapeutic action. These herbs have a very powerful effect and sometimes can be unsettling to the stomach and intestinal tract. The aromatic and carminative herbs will make the active herbs more palatable and settle the stomach and intestines. The aromatic and carminative herbs in these formulas usually stimulate digestion and circulation. In this way, they can actually make the active herbs more effective and more efficiently send the therapeutic agents to the sites in the body where they are needed. Such aromatic and carminative herbs include ginger, cayenne, cloves, and peppermint. The demulcent herbs will soothe the gastrointestinal tract. Since many disease conditions are a direct result of or associated with poor elimination and build-up of toxins, the cleansing herbs are used to improve elimination. However, the cleansing action in many of the formulas may be so gentle that it is hardly noticed except in overall improved health and sense of well-being.

CONCLUSION

The use of medicinal herbs dates back thousands of years. It is probably quite safe to say that every culture has used herbs medicinally. With the advent of modern medicine and the race of drug companies to patent new synthetic chemicals for profit, we have almost forgotten our roots. We often refer to modern medicine, as practiced in the United States, as conventional medicine. But we forget the fact that, by far, most of the world's population still successfully relies on herbal medicine. We like to tout our medical prowess, but the United States ranks behind more than 15 other countries in infant mortality. Perhaps the rest of the world continues to practice the true conventional medicine while we are on some modern medical experiment. Many Americans have become disenchanted with modern medicine and are finding great success with herbal medicine and other therapies. However, it is important to understand that no single philosophy of diagnosis and treatment contains all the answers. Nevertheless, I feel the answers will be more efficiently found as the various health care approaches are integrated than if they were to remain isolated and separate. I feel we can take the best of what we have learned in modern medicine and integrate with it alternative therapies for the betterment of the human family.

1

INFERTILITY

Indications:	Infertility, impotence, hot flashes, hormonal imbalances, menstrual problems
Recommended Formula:	Damiana leaves, ginseng root (Siberian), saw palmetto berries, kelp, sarsaparilla root, buckthorn bark
Dosage:	Three to six capsules daily. For chronic conditions it is best to use maximum dosage of six capsules per day for a prolonged period of two to three months. When adequate results have been achieved, cut dosage to three capsules daily.
Contraindications:	None
Doctor's Review:	This herbal formula is excellent for both men and women afflicted with infertility, impotence and other hormone imbalance related conditions. It does more than treat symptoms; it attacks the root of the problem returning the body to normal function. Its mode of action is both pharmacological and nutritive. Although the ancient Mayans used damiana leaves as an aphrodisiac and damiana maintains some of the same popularity today, this formula is not a magic potion of alluring aphrodisiacal properties or consequences. However, this formula is a serious remedy that will revitalize

reproductive and sexual function. It may also be used prophylactically to maintain good reproductive and sexual function and prevent degeneration of the same.

DOCTOR'S NOTES

Damiana Leaves:

Damiana's reputation began when it was discovered that native Mexican Indians used it for nervous and sexual debility and for mild constipation. The Indians also used damiana as a tonic and to soothe the gastrointestinal tract. Damiana now enjoys recognition in the *British Herbal Pharmacopeia* where it is reported to be a stimulant, mild diuretic, and a mild laxative. Germany's Commission E (the regulatory body that oversees phytomedicines) has published an official monograph on damiana suggesting it to be used as an aphrodisiac and for prophylaxis as well as a treatment for sexual disorders. Damiana seems to be particularly effective when combined with saw palmetto berries.

Siberian Ginseng:

Siberian ginseng, like damiana, has been popular for centuries as an aphrodisiac. It has probably enjoyed this reputation not because it stimulates sexual desire, but because it improves the health of the gastro-reproductive systems of the body. Thus, people who feel reproductively and sexually revitalized will have greater sexual performance and satisfaction. Stress, quite often, is a major causative factor of infertility and sexual dysfunction. Siberian ginseng has a clinically supported reputation as a stress fighter. It helps the body to cope with stress and maintain proper function.

Saw Palmetto Berries:

The saw palmetto berry has been popular among the American Indians of the South for treatment of urinary disorders. While the product has been listed in the *National Formulary*, it has become very popular in Europe as a treatment for benign prostate hypertrophy (BPH). In South America, it is used in combination with other herbs by women who find it to be more effective than prescription drugs for painful menstruation and pelvic congestion. Saw palmetto seems to exert a hormone balancing effect irrespective of gender.

Kelp:

Kelp performs three major functions in the herbal formula. First, it provides organic iodine for proper function of the thyroid gland. A dysfunctional thyroid gland can cause weakness, general malaise, and obesity. These conditions can contribute to lack of sexual desire and function. Second, it provides trace elements so often lacking in the American diet. Trace elements are co-factors in many metabolic processes of the body which can contribute to overall health. Third, it provides mucilage which helps to soothe the GI tract and maintain its proper function.

Sarsaparilla Root:

Sarsaparilla has a reputation as a fighter of syphilis and other venereal diseases. It also contains hormone precursors which help the body to maintain proper hormonal function. Sarsaparilla root is a diuretic as well as a reputed blood purifier helping to maintain general health.

Buckthorn Bark:

Buckthorn bark is included in this formula as an extremely mild laxative. Its effect is so subtle it may not be obvious. Stress and sexual debility may result in constipation. This could exacerbate lower abdominal pelvic congestion and compromise a sense of well being.

Other Supportive Nutrients

Dong quai, licorice root, angelica root, chaste tree berry, vitamin A, vitamin B-6, vitamin B-12, vitamin A, vitamin C, vitamin E, folic acid, niacin, pantothenic acid, calcium, magnesium, selenium, zinc, evening primrose oil, l-cysteine, l-arginine

2
ARTHRITIS

Indications:	Arthritis, rheumatism, bursitis, gout
Recommended Formula:	Devil's claw, yucca, alfalfa leaf and seed; wild yam root, sarsaparilla root, kelp, white willow bark, cayenne, horsetail, chickweed
Dosage:	Four to six capsules daily. For extreme cases it is best to use maximum dosage of six capsules per day for a prolonged period of four to six months.
Contraindications:	None
Doctor's Review:	A common problem many people have is generically referred to as rheumatism. Rheumatism includes different forms of arthritis such as osteoarthritis, muscle aches and pains, tendinitis, and fibromyositis. These conditions have a variety of underlying causes but have two elements in common. The first is inflammation, and the second, pain, is often a result of the first. This blend is designed to alleviate the symptoms of inflammation and pain and also to provide a rich nutrient base to help the body's healing process and return the body to normal function.

DOCTOR'S NOTES

Devil's Claw:	Don't let the name of this herb scare you off. It is so named because the plant's barbed hooks (claw)

when stepped on with bare feet, would "hurt like the devil," and you would have "a devil of a time getting them out of your feet." The secondary roots of this plant have a rich history of use as an anti-inflammatory, analgesic and digestive stimulant. There is probably no other herb with a greater reputation for treating rheumatism than devil's claw. It has gained official recognition as an antirheumatic and digestive agent in many European countries including France, Germany, Belgium, and Britain.

Because of its anti-inflammatory and analgesic properties, it is obvious how devil's claw would help with rheumatism. However, less evident is how its digestive stimulant properties can assist. Poor digestion usually results in greater putrefaction in the colon, consequently larger amounts of histamine are produced. Histamine triggers inflammation and therefore could exacerbate rheumatic conditions. A second consequence of poor digestion may be the absorption into the bloodstream of partially digested proteins called peptides. Sometimes the body considers peptides to be a foreign substance, or antigen, and in response produces antibodies or larger amounts of histamine. Some people have found that when they improve the health of their digestive system, rheumatic symptoms disappear.

Yucca: Yucca has a similar action to that of devil's claw. It improves digestion, thereby reducing histamine production and, as a result, inflammation and pain may be alleviated. The constituents of yucca commonly considered to be its actives are called saponins.

Alfalfa Leaves and Seeds: As mentioned in the previous two paragraphs, rheumatism may be a result of poor digestion. An impaired digestive system can cause malnutrition by starving the body of much needed macro- and micronutrients. If allowed to become chronic, serious and debilitating diseases can be the consequence. Alfalfa leaves and seeds provide a rich nutrient source to help the body to return to a healthy state.

Wild Yam Root: Other common names for wild yam root include rheumatism root and colic root, suggesting its use as an antirheumatic and digestive aid. Its antirheumatic property is primarily thought to be attributed to its cortisone precursor diosgenin. As diosgenin is converted to cortisone, anti-inflammatory activity results, and the patient may notice a reduction of pain. Also, wild yam root is a mild diuretic which helps to gently cleanse the body of toxins and waste, improving the body s internal environment and health.

Sarsaparilla Root: Sarsaparilla which is used as a food flavoring in the United States, is officially recognized in Germany and the United Kingdom for its antirheumatic, anti-inflammatory, and diuretic properties. Its activity is thought to be due to its saponin content. Historically, this herb has been used to treat gout and rheumatism and is classified as a tonic and blood purifier.

Kelp: Kelp, like alfalfa, is a dense source of nutrients, particularly trace elements which can improve the body's nutrition. It also provides mucilage in the form of algin which soothes the GI tract.

White Willow Bark: White willow bark has been used for over a thousand years to relieve pain. Salicin, aspirin's forerunner, was discovered to be white willow's active constituent. Apart from its ability to assist with pain, salicin reduces inflammation, but unlike aspirin it will not thin the blood or irritate the stomach.

Cayenne:

Cayenne stimulates circulation and makes the other herbs more effective. Cayenne can help to improve digestion. Cayenne's hot principle, capsaicin, is also a noted analgesic.

Horsetail (Shave Grass):

While horsetail contributes to this formula as a mild diuretic, its main action is to strengthen and regenerate connective tissues. Connective tissue (found abundantly in joints) is destroyed by inflammation. Silica is vital in regenerating connective tissue and keeping it strong. Horsetail is one of the richest known sources of silica.

Chickweed:

Chickweed supports the overall cleansing of the body by providing a mild laxative effect. The effect from this herb is so gentle that most people will not be aware of the action.

Other Supportive Nutrients

chamomile, ginseng, elecampane, astragalus, vitamin B-6, vitamin C, vitamin K, pantothenic acid, copper, selenium, zinc, omega-3 fatty acids (fish oils), evening primrose oil, dl-phenylalanine, l-cystine, bromelain, glycosaminoglycans, quercetin, superoxide dismutase, reduce dietary fat

3

RESPIRATORY DISTRESS

Indications:

Bronchitis, asthma, pneumonia, tuberculosis, cough, sore throat, colds, hayfever

Recommended Formula:

Pleurisy root, wild cherry bark, slippery elm bark, plantain, mullein leaves, chickweed, horehound, licorice root, kelp, ginger root, saw palmetto berries

Dosage:

Four to eight capsules daily. For chronic conditions it is best to use maximum dosage of eight capsules per day for a prolonged period of three to six weeks or until symptoms subside.

Contraindications:

None

Doctor's Review:

Respiratory distress can be caused by a wide variety of factors and can exhibit itself with many different symptoms. This formula is designed to ameliorate the symptoms and assist in overcoming some of the underlying causes. Herbs have been used for respiratory ailment by various cultures all over the world for thousands of years. There is strong historical documentation for these particular applications. Herbs are very effective, but one should not overlook the fact that they are also virtually free of side effects. Conventional drugs used to treat respiratory ailments are often riddled with side effects making the herbal approach even more attractive. This formula will help manage a wide range of problems, from asthma and bronchitis, to congestion, hoarseness, and sore throats.

DOCTOR'S NOTES

Pleurisy Root:

The English word *pleurisy* comes from the French word *pleurisis* which means, "lung trouble," indicating a primary use for this herb. Technically, pleurisy is an inflammatory condition affecting a thin lining covering the lungs and thorax and is usually a complication of pneumonia, tuberculosis, and other infectious diseases. This root has been used for other respiratory problems including bronchitis and catarrh. Pleurisy root also helps to cleanse the body of toxins through mild diuretic effects and its ability to promote perspiration.

Wild Cherry Bark:

Wild cherry bark has always been a favorite in cough and cold medicines. However, its most effective action benefits asthmatics by relaxing or sedating the respiratory nerves. Wild cherry bark also improves the stomach, digestion, and appetite which may provide a secondary healing benefit to people suffering respiratory ailments.

Slippery Elm Bark:

Slippery Elm bark has a reputation as a medicine for bronchitis, pleurisy and coughs. It has received official recognition in the *United States Pharmacopeia*. The inner bark is known for its demulcent, diuretic and emollient properties attributable to its high mucilage content. This bark is cleansing, healing, and strengthening and is particularly effective for inflammatory irritation associated with sore throats.

Plantain:

Plantain is similar to Slippery Elm bark in that it too contains mucilage. Plantain is used as an expectorant and is especially good for those suffering chronic catarrhal problems. It is also beneficial for hoarseness and sore throats. It seems to be able to help almost all respiratory problems.

Mullein Leaves:

Mullein leaves also contain high amounts of mucilage. While it is considered to be a good remedy for coughs, hoarseness, bronchitis, catarrh and whooping cough it stands out as an antispasmodic in treating asthma. Mullein leaves were officially recognized as an asthma treatment in the *National Formulary* until 1936.

Chickweed:

Chickweed is a folk remedy for asthma, but is also recognized as an expectorant. It has mild laxative effects which will contribute to the cleansing and healing process.

Horehound:

Horehound is an excellent remedy for coughs and bronchial problems. Its activity is thought to be attributed to a volatile oil found in the herb called *marubiin*. Horehound helps to cleanse the body of toxins through its diuretic properties and ability to promote perspiration.

Licorice Root:

Licorice root has received official recognition in Britain, Germany, France, and Belgium for its ability to assist with various respiratory problems which include bronchitis, hoarseness, coughs, sore throats, catarrh, and congestion. It shares some of the same properties as other herbs of this formula in cleansing and healing through its mild diuretic and laxative properties.

Kelp:

Kelp's direct application in this formula is in assisting with bronchitis, emphysema, and asthma. However, indirectly kelp provides a very rich storehouse of nutrients which can assist with the healing process.

Ginger Root:

Ginger root makes the other herbs more effective. Ginger is also an antispasmodic, and assists with coughs.

Saw Palmetto Berries:

Saw palmetto berries are useful in the treatment of colds, asthma, bronchitis and catarrhal problems. The berries are recognized for their diuretic properties, thereby contributing to the overall cleansing action of this formula.

Other Supportive Nutrients

Ginkgo biloba, ephedra, lobelia, echinacea, goldenseal root, elderberry flower, vitamin A, vitamin B-6, vitamin B-12, vitamin C, vitamin D, vitamin E, choline, inositol, pantothenic acid, calcium, magnesium, potassium, zinc, unsaturated fatty acids, bioflavonoids, water

4

SKIN DISORDERS

Indications: Eczema, psoriasis, acne, rash

Recommended Formula: Burdock root, gotu kola, yellow dock, dandelion root, milk thistle seeds, Irish moss, red clover blossoms, kelp, cayenne, sarsaparilla

Dosage: Two to six capsules daily. For chronic conditions use maximum dosage of six capsules per day for a prolonged period. For best results use every day.

Contraindications: None

Doctor's Review: The skin is the largest and one of the most important organs of the body. It performs many vital functions including cleansing toxic substances from the body, keeping the body's temperature in check and providing a barrier to pathogenic bacteria and viruses. The condition of the skin is often a reflection of the health of the body. Imbalances and toxic build-up due to a dysfunctional liver or improper elimination may reveal themselves in the skin as eczema, psoriasis, rashes, acne, dermatitis, or a number of other disorders. By improving the internal health of the body, the skin's functionality and appearance will be positively affected.

This formula is designed to cleanse the body by activating all its methods of elimination which include cleansing, strengthening, and supporting liver function. This formula will assist with a wide range of skin disorders including eczema, cellulitis, acne, psoriasis, burns, and insect bites. Longer lasting and more wide ranging results can be achieved by improving the diet and abstaining from chocolate, nuts and stimulants such as caffeine.

DOCTOR'S NOTES

Burdock Root:

If there was ever an herb to promote healthy skin through internal cleansing, burdock is it. Burdock root's cleansing power is multifaceted. It has a diaphoretic action (promotes perspiration) which expels toxins from the skin and blood. It promotes liver function and increases bile flow, which in turn cleanses the blood and reduces toxin production in the GI tract. In addition, burdock root is a mild laxative and diuretic which action further cleanses toxins from the body and improves general health. Burdock root is officially recognized in Britain, France, Germany and Belgium for its internal cleansing properties and its ability to treat skin disorders.

Gotu Kola:

Even though this herb has a similar sounding name to a popular soft drink, it is not related to the kola nut nor does it contain any caffeine. Gotu kola is supported by tremendous clinical research performed in Europe. This research demonstrates that gotu kola is effective in the treatment of various skin disorders associated with cellulitis and lupus. It also possesses wound healing activity and has been shown to decrease scarring.

Yellow Dock:

Yellow dock root is a reputed blood purifier and has been prescribed for all types of skin problems including leprosy, boils, and eczema. It has also been reported to clear a congested liver. Its laxative effect is well documented and supports the body's detoxifying ability.

Dandelion Root:

The common yard weed dandelion has a long history of use in herbal medicine. It is part of this formula for its ability to strengthen the liver, improve bile formation, regulate the bowels, purify the blood, and tonify the skin.

Milk Thistle:

There is probably not a person alive who could not be benefited by milk thistle. This wonderful herb cleanses, strengthens, and protects the liver and its functions. Time tested and proven in hospitals and clinics all over Europe, milk thistle is one of the only herbs known to treat some forms of psoriasis.

Irish Moss:

The contribution of Irish moss is very simple. It provides a demulcent and soothing source of mucilage and improves intestinal function.

Red Clover Blossom:

Red clover blossoms are a reputed blood purifier and officially recognized in the United Kingdom for treatment of skin conditions such as psoriasis, eczema, and rashes.

Kelp:

Kelp serves a similar function as Irish moss, but kelp is thought to be a blood purifier with the ability to alleviate skin problems, burns, and insect bites.

Cayenne:

Cayenne is a stimulant that helps to make all the other herbs function better. Such herbs are referred to as activators.

Sarsaparilla Root:

Sarsaparilla root has many benefits including the treatment of psoriasis and eczema. As a result of its diuretic and diaphoretic action sarsaparilla cleanses the body. This herb has received official recognition in European countries.

Other Supportive Nutrients

Centella asiatica, myrrh gum spray (topical), aloe gel, elecampane, vitamin A, vitamin B-2, vitamin B-6, vitamin B-12, vitamin C, vitamin D, vitamin E, biotin, choline, folic acid, inositol, PABA, magnesium, selenium, sulfur, zinc, evening primrose oil, unsaturated fatty acids, lecithin, bioflavonoids, glycosaminoglycans

5
DIABETES

Indications:	High blood sugar, diabetes
Recommended Formula:	Uva-ursi, dandelion root, fenugreek seeds, gentian root, huckleberry leaves, parsley, raspberry leaves, saw palmetto berries, kelp, bladderwrack, buchu
Dosage:	Three to nine capsules daily. It is best to start at a lower dosage for two to three weeks and gradually increase until desired benefit is achieved.
Contraindications:	Hypoglycemia, nephritis, sodium rich diets, potassium deficient diets
Doctor's Review:	Diabetes is essentially a carbohydrate metabolism disorder for which the cause is still unknown. However, Western cultures consuming highly processed and refined foods have a significantly higher percentage of diabetics than cultures consuming a more primitive diet.
	Diabetes is a condition where beta cells of the pancreas fail to produce sufficient insulin. Beta cells are part of cell clusters found in the pancreas and are responsible for secreting insulin. Other factors such as a diseased, injured or inflamed pancreas as well as certain medications can also cause diabetes. Some

forms of diabetes require insulin while other forms can be controlled with the proper diet. Diabetes usually leads to vascular and neural disorders. For example, in advanced stages poor circulation can necessitate the amputation of a limb or cause blindness. Uncontrolled diabetes can initiate a diabetic coma or death. Diabetes is a progressive disease influenced by factors including obesity, diet, meal frequency and hygiene.

Diabetic or prediabetic persons should consult a health care professional and learn all the facts about diabetes. As one learns how to control the disease, frequent consultation with a physician is strongly suggested. This herbal formula is not a cure for diabetes. However, it is designed to support the body, especially the glands and organs which are prone to weakness and dysfunction in diabetics. This formula is a wonderful adjunct to the diabetic diet and therapies. This formula may reduce the insulin dose requirements in insulin-dependent diabetics; therefore, insulin dosage should be closely monitored when initiating this formula.

Doctor's Note:

Uva-Ursi: Uva-ursi is very popular, especially in Europe where it is found in most herbal teas designed to treat bladder and kidney disorders. Kidney disease is a major and common complication and a leading cause of death in diabetics. Therefore, kidney health is of prime concern to the diabetic. Uva-ursi has historically been used to treat kidney and bladder inflammatory diseases and infections. It tonifies the urinary passages and helps to prevent kidney stones.

Uva-ursi is a diuretic that helps cleanse toxins from the blood and expel them from the body. Two important compounds found in uva-ursi are arbutin and quercitin. Arbutin is converted to hydroquinone, a well recognized antiseptic for the urinary tract. Quercetin is a powerful aldose reductase (AR) inhibitor. AR is implicated in the formation of diabetic cataracts. Quercetin is an inhibitor of platelet aggregation which is the genesis of blood clots. Strokes can be caused by blood clots and are often often a complication of diabetes. Uva-ursi is officially recognized in Russia, Switzerland, France, Germany, and Britain.

Dandelion Root:

Dandelion root has many properties that influence general health. It improves digestion by stimulating bile production, improves liver function, removes excess fluids from the body, improves circulation and strengthens weak arteries. Dandelion root has a mild laxative effect which further cleanses the body.

Fenugreek Seeds:

Scientific studies have demonstrated that fenugreek seeds have an anti-diabetic effect. Consistent intake of seeds stimulates pancreatic function. Fenugreek seeds contain a soothing mucilaginous material that improves GI tract function.

Gentian Root:

Gentian root is one of the most popular bitter tonics in Europe. It is used to help with all digestive disorders. Gentian strengthens the pancreas and tonifies the spleen and kidneys.

Huckleberry Leaves:

Huckleberry is a close relative of uva-ursi and exhibits many of the same properties. Huckleberry is believed to contain a natural insulin compound which assists in blood sugar control.

Parsley:

Parsley has a long history of use as a medicine, particularly in Europe. While it is a wonderful tonic herb, its main application in this formula is its effect on urinary tract health. Parsley also assists in maintaining the health of other organs like the liver and spleen. Parsley's carminative action makes it a popular garnish at meal times.

Raspberry Leaves:

Raspberry leaves are one of the best herbal remedies for diarrhea. Occasionally diarrhea is caused by autonomic neuropathy (a disorder of the part of the nervous system responsible for involuntary bodily functions) present with diabetes. This condition is also responsible for tachycardia and other cardiovascular problems which may be helped by raspberry leaves since they are considered to be cardiotonic. Raspberry leaves are also astringent and have been used to treat lesions, wounds, and ulcers which often plague the diabetic.

Saw Palmetto Berries:

A tremendous amount of scientific research has scrutinized saw palmetto berries. Saw palmetto berries have been proven effective for benign prostate enlargement. Prostate inflammation, usually in advanced cases, can trigger kidney problems by not allowing the elimination of urine. It also seems to assert a hormone balancing effect on both men and women which may contribute to overall well-being.

Kelp:

Kelp's high level of micro nutrients assists in many of the body's metabolic processes. The high iodine content will help with thyroid function and in turn with weight control. Obesity can create many problems for the diabetic. Kelp further improves health by providing a soothing algin to the GI tract.

Bladderwrack:

Bladderwrack is part of the kelp family and contains many of the same important compounds and elements found in kelp. Germany, France, and Britain recognize Bladdewrack for its ability to fight obesity and hypothyroidism.

Buchu Leaves:

Buchu was listed in the *National Formulary* years ago for the treatment of urinary tract disorders. In the mid-1800s buchu was often sold as a treatment for diabetes and various kidney problems. Buchu is still popular in France, Germany, and Britain for maintaining urinary tract health.

Other Supportive Nutrients

Ginkgo biloba, bilberry, ginseng, gymnema sylvestre, bitter melon, beta carotene, vitamin B-1, vitamin B-12, vitamin C, vitamin D, vitamin E, biotin, inositol, niacin, pantothenic acid, calcium, chromium, copper, magnesium, manganese, phosphorus, potassium, zinc, evening primrose oil, lecithin, glutathione, bioflavonoids, coenzyme Q10, quercitin, inulin, brewers yeast, fiber, complex carbohydrate

6
WATER RETENTION

Indications:	Water retention or edema, dropsy, cystitis, gout
Recommended Formula:	Cornsilk, parsley, uva-ursi, cleavers, juniper berries, kelp, cayenne, queen of the meadow, buchu
Dosage:	Two to eight capsules daily. Should not be used continuously. ´
Contraindications:	Kidney dysfunction, nephritis, pregnancy
Doctor's Review:	Water retention is a common problem, but its causes can be quite diverse. Electrolyte imbalances, excessive capillary permeability, increased capillary pressure, heart failure, liver and renal dysfunction, and chemical substances such as: venoms, toxins, and histamine can all cause water retention.
	Water retention can be so mild that it is hardly noticeable or it can be morbidly pronounced as exhibited in dropsy. In modern society many people, especially women, are more concerned with the cosmetic effects of water retention. Some people go to great lengths to expel excess water so they may appear thinner. However, there is a danger in the long-term use of diuretics which can cause electrolyte imbalances, particularly a deficiency in potassium.

When using diuretics for more than a few days at a time, a diet rich in potassium or potassium supplementation should be observed. Also, long term use of diuretics can place excessive hardship on the kidneys. This formula contains herbs that have a long history of use in treating water retention. In conjunction with this herbal treatment one should reduce or restrict sodium (salt) and fluid intake. Bed rest may also be beneficial.

DOCTOR'S NOTES

Cornsilk:

Cornsilk's benefits for the urinary tract and in the treatment of water retention are well acknowledged. Cornsilk is found on every continent except Antarctica. Europeans have been using it for centuries as a diuretic to fight urinary infections and as a urinary demulcent. Today cornsilk has gained official recognition in France, Britain, and Belgium.

Parsley:

Parsley is another herb well utilized for its medicinal value in Europe. It is used in Britain and Germany as a diuretic; however, particularly in Germany, it is used to provide irrigation in treating kidney stones. The main constituents thought to provide this diuretic action are myristicin and apiole. Parsley provides a carminative action which is one reason for its popularity as a garnish at meal time.

Uva-Ursi:

Uva-ursi is one of the best researched diuretics obtained from the plant kingdom. Its urinary tract applications extend far beyond diuresis, urethritis, cystitis, and other urinary inflammatory diseases. Urinary bacterial infections are ameliorated by uva-ursi. It contains arbuti which is converted to hydroquinone in t body, producing antiseptic properties for t urinary tract. Uva-ursi is officially recognized many countries including Russia, Switzerlan France, Germany, and Britain.

Cleavers:

Cleavers is considered by some herbalists to l one of the best herbs for kidney and bladd troubles. It is especially good for cases of kidn stones and water retention. It is also benefici for painful urination. It provides a mild laxati effect, further cleansing the body and returni it to a more normal state of health.

Juniper Berries:

Juniper berries are just one more weapo against urinary tract disorders and wat retention found in this herbal formula's arsen: Juniper is particularly effective at expelling u acid which is associated with stone formation the kidneys.

Kelp:

Kelp exhibits only mild diuretic activity, but i real application to this blend is its ability replace trace elements that are lost throug urination. Trace element imbalances and lo are a major problem with extended diurect use. Kelp also contains algin which provides mild laxative effect and a soothing demulce to the GI tract.

Cayenne:

Cayenne is a great circulation stimulan Increased circulation causes more blood to flo into the glomeruli of the kidney which w release more fluid as urine. Therefore, cayeni has an indirect diuretic effect. Cayenne will al improve the effectiveness of the other herbs.

ueen of the Meadow Root:	Also known as kidney root and gravel root, these names give a glimpse of queen of the meadow root's applications. It is used as a diuretic and to treat chronic urinary disorders, dropsy and kidney stones.
uchu Leaves:	Buchu leaves are said to be able to absorb excess uric acid and be soothing to the organs of the urinary tract. They have been used to treat conditions where there has been a stoppage of urine. They are also beneficial in cases of prostate enlargement.

Other Supportive Nutrients

Bladderwrack, artichoke, burdock root, vitamin B-1, vitamin B-6, vitamin C, vitamin D, vitamin E, pantothenic acid, calcium, copper, potassium, protein, reduce sodium

7

FEMALE DISORDERS

FORMULA A:
YEAST INFECTIONS

Indications:	Vaginal yeast infections or vaginitis.
Recommended Formula:	Goldenseal root, witch hazel leaves, plantain myrrh gum, pau d'arco, slippery elm bark, blu cohosh root, uva-ursi leaves, juniper berries.
Dosage:	Four to eight capsules daily. For chroni conditions it is best to use maximum dosage o eight capsules per day for prolonged period o four to six weeks or until symptoms are gone However, it should not be used for more thar three months without at least a two-week break
Contraindications:	None
Doctor's Review:	Vaginitis or more particularly vaginal yeas infections are a growing problem in America today. One of the contributing factors is the widespread use of antibiotic therapy for sucl things as urinary tract infections, colds, sore throats, eye infections, etc. Some women who contract a vaginal yeast infection after the use o antibiotic therapy quite often conclude that the yeast infection was much worse than the condition for which they used the antibiotics.

Many areas of the body, such as the gastrointestinal tract and the vaginal canal, are covered by a thin mucus lining. This mucus lining serves as a defense mechanism to keep bacteria, yeasts and viruses from being able to reach vulnerable tissues and cells. Antibiotic therapy can cause a disruption in the normal flora that exists in the body, not only in the gastrointestinal tract but also in the vaginal canal, allowing yeast to grow unchecked which can cause a disruption of the mucus lining. With the lining disrupted unhealthy organisms are better able to attack the tissues. Another significant factor could be a diet rich in refined carbohydrates which tends to lower the immune response and produce an environment conducive to yeast growth. This herbal formula helps to fight yeast infection and also helps to restore the mucus lining in the vaginal canal.

DOCTOR'S NOTES

Goldenseal Root:

Goldenseal root has a long history of use with bacterial infection, yeast infections and particularly vaginitis. Goldenseal root exerts a positive effect upon the mucus lining by creating stronger cross links between the mucosal proteins, making it much more difficult to disrupt the protective lining. Apart from its specific activity with vaginal yeast infections, goldenseal root is considered by many herbalists to be a very powerful tonic. It enjoys official recognition in France and Britain.

Witch Hazel Leaves:

For many years witch hazel leaves have been lauded by natural doctors and herbalists for their astringent and anti-inflammatory properties. Vaginal yeast can produce inflammation and irritation which often resul in the common symptom of itchiness. Witc hazel leaves provide symptomatic relief b reducing inflammation as well as itchiness.

A secondary benefit of witch hazel leaves their ability to shrink the blood vessels that a near the surface of the vaginal wall, preventir the yeast from penetrating the capillaries ar reducing the chance of bleeding. Witch haz leaves also seem to have an ability to maintai the integrity of the mucosal lining. Witch haz leaves are recommended by numerous docto and clinics all over the world and are officia recognized in the *British Herbal Pharmacopeia.*

Plantain:

Although plantain is not as well known as wit hazel leaves, it has been used in much the san way, providing similar benefits. In fact, wit hazel and plantain enjoy a common bor because they both have been used together formulas to help with hemorrhoids, bleedin inflammation and irritation. The *British Herk Pharmacopeia* is an example of a publicatio that recommends both witch hazel and planta be used together. Plantain's diuretic action hel to return the body to a more normal state health, and its mucilage content soothes t gastrointestinal tract.

Myrrh Gum:

Even before its use here in America, myrrh gu was highly valued in Africa, Europe and Chir Myrrh gum provides a powerful antisept action, particularly with mucous membran such as those which line the vaginal can; Myrrh gum has demonstrated an ability to effective at maintaining a healthy muco membrane and is said to be a good an inflammatory. Myrrh gum is also said to possess a mild laxative effect. This helps with the elimination of toxins produced by the yeast and speeds recovery of health.

au d' Arco: *Lapacho* and *ipe roxo* are other names by which pau d'arco is referred. Pau d' arco, a tree which grows up to 125 feet tall, is native to Brazil and other South American countries. It has been used by the native people of South America for hundreds if not thousands of years. Its benefits have to do with its antimicrobial properties. The constituents of pau d'arco which provide this benefit are a class of compounds called naphthoquinones. These naphthoquinones are highly effective against candida albicans, the perpetrator of vaginal yeast infections. Pau d' arco has demonstrated clear anti-inflammatory activity, especially with vaginal inflammation. Several dozen scientific studies acknowledge the helpful benefits of pau d' arco.

ippery Elm: Slippery elm has benefits much the same as witch hazel leaves and plantain leaves. However, slippery elm's action is more directed toward maintaining a healthy mucous lining. Slippery elm's benefits include healing and restoration. It soothes the gastrointestinal tract, helping it return to a more normal state of health. Slippery elm also helps to absorb and eliminate toxins from the body. It alleviates vaginal irritations and itching. Its many health benefits are officially recognized in the United States and in Great Britain, where it is found in over-the-counter medications.

lue Cohosh: Blue cohosh has a multitude of applications for the various elements that affect women. It is no wonder then why blue cohosh root has bee referred to as papoose root and squaw root. I various applications include bladder infection menstrual cramps, menstrual regulatio neuralgia, leucorrhea, pregnancy disorder spasms, and vaginitis. Its ability to help wii vaginitis is due to its antimicrobial property ar indirectly to its soothing effect on the nerves.

Uva-Ursi:

Uva-ursi has been used all over the world as diuretic. However, scientific studies ha demonstrated that a constituent in Uva-ur called arbutin is responsible for uva-urs antiseptic properties, with particular applicatio for the urinary tract. It has been used I herbalists to help in conditions of vaginitis ar vaginal yeast infections. Uva-ursi has gaine official recognition in Britain, Franc Germany, Sweden, and the USSR. Scientit studies have been performed in Russi Germany, France, Poland, and the form Czechoslovakia. Uva-ursi constitutes one of t most documented herbal medicines of today.

Juniper Berries:

Juniper berries and myrrh gum provi carminative and aromatic activity whi stimulates digestion and circulation. This w help the various herbs within this formula to more effective and be transported througho the body to the areas where they will utilized. Juniper berries in conjunction wi uva-ursi provide diuretic activity to reduce t overall congestion of the pelvic region. Junip berries play a supporting role in this formula.

Other Supportive Nutrients

Phellodendron (huang bai), vitamins A and vitamin B-complex, acidophilus, caprylic acid

FORMULA B:
EXCESSIVE MENSTRUAL FLOW

Indications: Excessive menstrual flow (menorrhagia, menorrhea)

Recommended Formula: Cranesbill, witch hazel leaves, red raspberry leaves, shepherd's purse, ginger root, horsetail, goldenseal root, Irish moss

Dosage: Four to six capsules daily. For chronic conditions it is best to use the maximum dosage of six capsules per day for a prolonged period of two to three months. When adequate results have been achieved cut dosage to four capsules daily.

Contraindications: None

Doctor's Review: Menorrhea and its synonym menorrhagia are words used to describe a condition of excessive bleeding at the time of a menstrual period. Profuse or excessive bleeding can be caused by a number of different factors including hormonal disturbances and systemic conditions such as diabetes mellitus, hypertension, and chronic nephritis, etc. The two properties that stand out most among the various herbs of this formula are the astringent and anti-hemorrhage properties. This formula is ideal for slowing down the loss of blood and preventing anemic conditions that can occur as a result of excessive blood loss. This combination of herbs can help with some of the underlying causes of menorrhagia—shepherd's purse with hypertension and cranesbill with diabetes. Excessive blood loss might indicate a more

serious condition where wisdom should dictat
that one seek the advice of a health car
professional.

Doctor's Notes

Cranesbill:

Cranesbill is considered by many herbalists t
possess a powerful astringent effect, whicl
means it will have a profound ability to shrin
or constrict tissue. The obvious result is
reduction in blood flow and prevention o
hemorrhage. This property has wide rangin;
benefits from troublesome nose bleeding t
hemorrhoids to menorrhea. Cranesbill is
diuretic which helps to cleanse impurities fron
the body and assist the body to function in
more normal way.

Witch Hazel Leaves:

Witch hazel has a rich history of use as a
astringent, anti-hemorrhagic and anti
inflammatory. It was listed in the *Nationa
Formulary* until 1955. It is still used today i
over-the-counter medications by larg
pharmaceutical companies like Parke-Davis. I
continues to have full acceptance and officia
recognition in Great Britain. Witch hazel help
to shrink inflamed or otherwise swollen bloo
vessels.

Red Raspberry Leaves:

A favorite among midwives, red raspberry leave
have a long history of use for various female
complaints before, during, and after pregnancy
Its direct contribution to this formula is due t
its astringent properties.

Shepherd's Purse:

Shepherd's purse originated in Europe but ha
since been naturalized all over the world. Many
cultures have used and incorporated it int

their traditional medicines. It has been used for thousands of years and was known as a medicine to the ancient Romans and Greeks. It retained much of its popularity in Europe throughout the Middle Ages but shortly thereafter fell into disuse. It wasn't until this century that there has been a revival of shepherd's purse, which has received official recognition in the *British Herbal Pharmacopeia* where it is noted for its astringent and diuretic properties. Shepherd's also purse works with the other astringent herbs of this formula to control bleeding, especially internal hemorrhaging. Its diuretic effect provides gentle cleansing, helping the body to restore health and normal function.

Ginger Root:

Even though ginger root was used by the eclectic physicians of the early 20th century for painful menstruation and other menstrual problems, its main contribution to this formula has to do with its aromatic, carminative and activating properties. This gives ginger the ability to improve digestion as well as bowel regularity and function, and also to stimulate circulation, helping to deliver the active astringent properties where they can be utilized.

Horsetail (Shave Grass):

Horsetail has, like other herbs of this formula, a long history of use, particularly as an astringent and also as a diuretic. It helps to prevent excessive bleeding and hemorrhage. It is officially recognized in a number of the European pharmacopeias. Horsetail's clinical use has been well accepted and documented. A recent animal study in Germany has confirmed its astringent properties. Horsetail also seems to follow the pattern of other strong powerful astringent herbs in that it has a diuretic effect,

gently cleansing the body and helping to restor
normal function and health.

Goldenseal Root:

Goldenseal root has many uses pertinent to th
formula. It has the ability to help wit
menorrhagia, post-partum hemorrhage an
dysmenorrhea. It is officially recognized in tw
pharmacopeias in Europe. Goldenseal root ha
another function worthy of note, particularly a
it applies to this formula. It has antimicrobi
properties. Any time there is hemorrhage, ther
is a propensity for infection. Goldenseal roc
may help to prevent mild or even seriou
infections if a hemorrhage does occur.

As a note of interest, goldenseal root wa
employed by the Russians during World War I
to help stop bleeding. When they were n
longer able to obtain goldenseal root fror
Canada and the United States where it grow
naturally, they resorted to another herb alread
mentioned in this formula, shepherd's purse. A
a final note, goldenseal root has been used as
mild laxative. This laxative effect cleanses th
body of toxins and impurities allowing for
better state of health.

Irish Moss:

Irish moss contributes mucilage to this formul
which soothes the gastrointestinal tract an
counteracts some of the negative effects tha
may occur due to the more powerful bitte
astringent herbs in this formula.

Other Supportive Nutrients

milk thistle, vitamin A, vitamin C, iror
vitamin E, iodine, bioflavonoids, formul
described in chapter 7C

FORMULA C:
FEMALE TONIC

Indications: Female tonic, difficult or painful menstruation, menopause

Recommended Formula: Black cohosh root, dong quai, passion flower, red raspberry leaves, fenugreek seeds, licorice root, chamomile, black haw bark, saw palmetto berries, wild yam root, kelp, butternut root bark

Dosage: Four to six capsules daily. For chronic conditions and imbalances maximum dosage of six capsules per day should be taken for several months or until normal function is restored. Best if used daily throughout the month.

Contraindications: Consult a health care professional before using this formula if you are pregnant or lactating.

Doctor's Review: One of the most common causes of female symptoms seems to center around hormone dysfunction. There are women who start having symptoms related to hormone fluctuation at menarche, the beginning of menstrual flow, right up to those who begin having symptoms only after menopause, the cessation of menstrual flow. There are also women who will live their entire lives without any symptoms related to hormone fluctuations. Then there are those who seem to be incessantly plagued by continually revolving symptoms surrounding hormone function and dysfunction.

This formula is specially designed to help modulate and decrease, or eliminate symptoms associated with hormone fluctuation and dysfunction. This formula incorporates other herbs that will allay symptoms of anxiety and painful cramping. Most women with the above related conditions would greatly benefit from consistent use of this particular formula.

DOCTOR'S NOTES

Black Cohosh Root:

Black cohosh root was so highly valued by the American Indian for female disorders that it was named "squaw root." Today black cohosh has been proven to be such an effective remedy for painful menstrual cramps, dysmenorrhea menopausal disorders and premenstrual complaints that it has received official recognition in Britain and Germany. Studies have shown black cohosh root to have endocrine activity with the ability to mimic estrogen. At one time black cohosh root enjoyed official recognition in the *National Formulary.* Antispasmodic and diuretic actions are other properties which contribute to the herb's usefulness in this formula.

Dong Quai:

There is no other herb used more widely in Chinese medicine for treatment of gynecological ailments than dong quai. Dong quai relieves menstrual cramps, corrects irregular or retarded menstrual flow, and alleviates unpleasant symptoms associated with menopause. Dong quai is said to have analgesic properties but this is probably due, in part, to its antispasmodic effect. As a side note, dong quai has been used to treat anemia which can result from excessive blood loss during menstruation. Because of dong quai's mild laxative effect, it has an ability to prevent an overall feeling of pelvic and abdominal congestion by assisting with elimination.

Passion Flower:

Many women experience anxiety prior to and during menses, and discomforts such as hot flashes when adjusting to menopause. Passion flower contributes a sedative action for anxiety and relieves spasms and cramps. It has an overall calming effect.

Red Raspberry Leaves:

Red raspberry leaves have long been used for various female afflictions during pregnancy and child birth in addition to those associated with menses. More specifically it strengthens and tonifies the uterus, stops hemorrhages, decreases excess and increases deficient menstrual flow, and relieves painful menstruation by relaxing the smooth muscles.

Fenugreek Seeds:

Although fenugreek seed has been used to assist proper menstruation and promote lactation, its main role in this formula stems from its other properties. Fenugreek is a tonic, mild diuretic, and a source for mucilage which provides soothing demulcent properties. Like many other seeds, fenugreek is nutritious and restorative, strengthening those recovering from illness or imbalances.

Licorice Root:

Licorice root is incorporated into about a third of all Chinese herbal formulas and a majority of the formulas dealing with female reproductive problems. This is an indication that it has tremendous versatility. Indeed, licorice supports the effects of all the other herbs of the formula. Perhaps, this is the main reason the Chinese call it the "Great Adjunct." Licorice not only contains hormonal precursors but stimulates the production of estrogen. This has been shown to decrease the symptoms associated with hormone fluctuation. It is also prized for

its demulcent and mild laxative properti❙
Licorice root has received official recognition
Britain, Belgium, France and Germany.
many countries it is recognized for its an❙
inflammatory and antispasmodic properti
suggesting more ways in which licori❙
contributes to this formula.

Chamomile:

Aside from chamomile's carminative and ton❙
properties, this herb has gained wor❙
recognition for its anodyne (pain relieving
antispasmodic, and antianxiety propertie
Chamomile has demonstrated its worth ❙
many clinical studies, officially monographed
Britain, Belgium, France, and Germany.

Black Haw Bark:

Another name for black haw bark is cramp ba❙
suggesting the reason for its inclusion in th❙
formula. Historical and folkloric use as well
scientific evidence have proven this bark to ❙
effective against muscle spasms and menstru❙
dysfunction, especially inconsistent estrus cycle

Saw Palmetto Berries:

Saw palmetto berries have been used ❙
American Indians for hundreds of years. Tod❙
this herb has been scientifically and clinical❙
proven effective for male and fema
genitourinary problems. One study has show
it to be many times more effective tha❙
prescription anti-inflammatory medication ❙
the treatment of pelvic congestion associate
with menstrual dysfunction. As an interestin❙
side note, saw palmetto can prevent the grow❙
of unwanted facial hair in women.

Wild Yam Root:

Wild yam root contains the steroidal sapone❙
botogenin and *diosgenin.* These are precursors ❙
cortisone and other hormones. Wild yam h❙

antispasmodic effects and is soothing to the nerves. It is also diuretic and helps to eliminate painful urination. It is highly recommended for cramping.

Kelp: Kelp provides important trace elements which are often missing or deficient in Western diets. Trace elements assist with many metabolic processes in the body, without which may lead to various problems. Kelp contains algin which provides soothing benefits to the GI tract.

Butternut Root Bark: Butternut is a soothing laxative which helps to restore general health and sense of well-being. Its laxative effect in this formula may be too gentle for it to be obvious.

Other Supportive Nutrients

vitamin B-6, vitamin C, vitamin D, vitamin E, niacin, calcium, iodine, magnesium, potassium, evening primrose oil, protein, formula described in chapter 7B

8

HEART TROUBLE

Indications:	Weak heart muscle, arrhythmia, angina, shortness of breath, palpitations
Recommended formula:	Hawthorn berries, motherwort, rosemary leaves, cayenne, kelp, wood betony, shepherd's purse
Dosage:	Four to six capsules daily. May be used daily.
Contraindications:	None
Doctor's Review:	The average heart beats over one hundred thousand times a day and about 38 million times per year. To illustrate, this remarkable organ raises the equivalent of one ton to a height of 41 feet every 24 hours. The heart muscle must beat 24 hours a day to sustain life. Heart defects can be of various origins. Some are inborn errors; others are caused by aging, disease, or illness, such as rheumatic fever and beriberi. Fortunately there are many herbs which support the function of the heart.

The highly effective heart medicine "digitalis" is actually a derivative of a botanical commonly known as fox glove or *Digitalis purpurea*. While digitalis is associated with a narrow safety margin and not found in this formula, many other botanicals described hereafter are quite safe and effective. This formula can strengthen a weak heart, restore proper heart rhythm, reduce blood pressure and prevent angina.

DOCTOR'S NOTES

Hawthorn Berry:

Next to digitalis, hawthorn is probably the most recognized herb for positively affecting the heart. As demonstrated by scientific studies, hawthorn supports metabolic processes in the heart, dilates coronary vessels, reduces peripheral resistance and lowers blood pressure, reduces tendency for angina attacks and strengthens damaged or weakened heart muscles. Hawthorn is found in many European herbal calming formulas which suggests an effect on the central nervous system. This may help when heart problems are caused by stress or anxiety. The *British Herbal Pharmacopeia* indicates hawthorn is reputed to dissolve deposits in sclerotic arteries. Hawthorn is perhaps the best cardiotonic known today.

Motherwort:

No heart formula would be complete without motherwort. The use of motherwort as a cardiotonic spans centuries. Its other common names such as *heart heal* and *heart wort* are more indicative of its heart benefits than the appellation *motherwort.* Nevertheless it has been proven worthy for official recognition in Britain, Germany, and France. Motherwort is especially beneficial in cases of nervous heart conditions which can cause, among other things, palpitation or abnormally rapid or fluttering heart beats. Motherwort normalizes the heart in at least two ways. It asserts a calming action on the central nervous system which can help to normalize heart rate, and it assists in improving thyroid function in cases of hyperactivity. Hyperthyroidism is often associated with heart palpitation. The British recognize motherwort's ability to reduce blood pressure, and like hawthorn, it has a mild sedative action.

Rosemary Leaves:

Like many spices rosemary contains powerful antioxidants. Antioxidants have clearly been shown to support the integrity of the veins. Rosemary has also exhibited cardiotonic capacity which helps with normal heart function. Rosemary stimulates bile flow which improves digestion. It also causes mild perspiration, releasing toxins from the body and improving health.

Cayenne:

Cayenne supports and improves circulation. Cayenne is considered an herb activator that increases the effectiveness of other herbs. It stimulates digestion and promotes perspiration. Cayenne has been shown to reduce blood pressure, especially in conjunction with garlic.

Kelp:

Kelp is a powerhouse of micronutrients that assist with various metabolic processes. Kelp has been considered a blood vessel cleanser and a treatment for atherosclerosis. Kelp contains algin which is a soluble fiber that improves bowel function and soothes the GI tract. Kelp has also been suggested in cases of obesity and digestive problems.

Wood Betony:

Wood betony is carminative, diuretic, and nervine. The three benefits support a healthy cardiovascular system.

Shepherd's Purse:

Shepherd's purse is a common weed that grows all over the United States. It is diuretic and has an ability to regulate blood pressure and heart action.

Other Supportive Nutrients

goldenseal root, ginkgo biloba, valerian root, lobelia, vitamin A, carotene, vitamin B-complex, vitamin C, vitamin E, calcium, chromium, copper, magnesium, manganese, phosphorous, potassium, selenium, zinc, evening primrose oil, unsaturated fatty acid, lecithin, l-carnitine, taurine, coenzyme Q10

9

HIGH BLOOD PRESSURE

Indications:

High blood pressure (hypertension), high cholesterol

Recommended Formula:

Garlic, valerian root, black cohosh root, cayenne, kelp, blessed thistle, parsley leaves

Dosage:

Four to eight capsules daily. After an adequate reduction of blood pressure is achieved slowly reduce dosage while maintaining the effect.

Contraindications:

Pregnancy, lactation

Doctor's Review:

High blood pressure is not as easy to diagnose as it appears. To illustrate, some people will experience temporary elevation in blood pressure merely because of the anxiety generated when being diagnosed. Also there is still some controversy over what is considered to be high blood pressure. Nevertheless, high blood pressure can lead to other debilitating, or even deadly conditions and therefore should be taken seriously. Its causes can vary from psychogenic, to narrowing of blood vessels, to hyperthyroidism and kidney diseases, etc.

This formula contains herbs which have a rich history and scientifically supported use in conditions of high blood pressure. Some of the herbs will immediately begin to lower the pressure and at the same time work on the underlying cause. Garlic, or a combination of garlic and cayenne, has been used to reduce blood pressure, but this may not be as effective against some of the root causes as the other herbs found in this preferred formula. Lifestyle changes can also help. It is best to cut out tobacco, alcohol, and caffeine and to exercise according to the advice of a health care professional.

DOCTOR'S NOTES

Garlic:

Garlic has many different applications, but one that stands out is its ability to reduce blood pressure. Garlic also lowers triglycerides, cholesterol and lipoproteins found in the blood which reduce the risk of arteriosclerosis. Garlic is so effective it remains one of the most used herbs in the world including the western world. Garlic also contains compounds which inhibit platelet aggregation helping to prevent stroke. Strokes are often related to high blood pressure.

Valerian Root:

Valerian root is particularly beneficial for stress-induced hypertension. Valerian will calm and relax an anxious person. Valerian has the ability to reduce arrhythmia (irregular heart beats), and dilate blood vessels. The actives include valepotriates and valeric acid.

Black Cohosh Root:

Compounds like actein have been isolated from black cohosh and have been demonstrated to lower blood pressure in some animals. However, black cohosh has been recognized for years by herbalists to calm the cardiovascular system. Its diuretic and diaphoretic effects help to expel excess fluids from the body and assist in keeping the blood healthier.

Cayenne:

Cayenne has been used extensively and successfully with garlic in effecting a lower blood pressure. Cayenne is considered to be a blood pressure normalizer or adaptogen. It raises blood pressure that is too low and lowers blood pressure that is too high. Cayenne also serves to stimulate sluggish circulation and makes the other herbs of this formula work faster and better.

Kelp:

Kelp is a storehouse of nutrients which assist in maintaining various metabolic processes of the body and provides for improved nutrition. Kelp has been employed in Japanese medicine to keep blood pressure under control. Kelp also provides soluble fiber in the form of algin improving GI tract health and mildly stimulating bowel function.

Blessed Thistle:

Blessed thistle is considered a tonic herb which helps to improve general health. It enhances digestion by correcting liver and gall bladder disorders. It is also diuretic and promotes perspiration.

Parsley Leaves:

Parsley is used extensively in Europe as a diuretic and antispasm medicine. It is considered to be one of the more nutritious herbs. Apiole is a chemical constituent of parsley that helps to dilate blood vessels, which aids in reducing high blood pressure.

Other Supportive Nutrients

onion, hawthorn berry, lavender, vitamin A, vitamin B-complex, vitamin C, vitamin D, calcium, chromium, magnesium, potassium, zinc, evening primrose oil, flax seed oil, omega-3 and omega 6 fatty acids, lecithin, coenzyme Q10, chromium

10
PAIN

Indications:	Headache, migraine, arthritis pain, pain caused by inflammation, back ache, spasms, and fever
Recommended Formula:	White willow bark, blue vervain, feverfew leaves, rosemary leaves, skullcap, and kelp
Dosage:	Three to five capsules daily. May be used daily.
Contraindications:	Pregnancy

Doctor's Review:

Pain is a sensation most people will go to great lengths to avoid. It can, of course, vary in intensity from mild to severe, and is almost always associated with inflammation. Pain should be considered a message that something is wrong with some particular part of the body and needs to be corrected. The source of chronic pain should be properly diagnosed by a health care professional.

Many sources of pain can easily be fixed and the pain alleviated. This formula contains herbs that can assist in correcting the underlying cause of pain. Some herbs can perform well where prescription medications have failed. While this herb formula has its limitations with regard to intense pain, its applications are quite broad.

DOCTOR'S NOTES

White Willow:

White willow bark has been used for thousands of years to help relieve pain. The bark contains a substance called salicin which is believed by some to convert to salicylic acid, or aspirin in the body. While they both help with pain, salicin, unlike aspirin, does not thin the blood or irritate the stomach. For this reason some people believe that salicin is not converted to aspirin in the body, but that its pain relieving mechanism may be due to something else. In either case, white willow is a natural and effective herb for pain relief. White willow can reduce fever and inflammation, and is particularly useful in treating articular rheumatism. White willow's diuretic and diaphoretic properties will provide for improved health as toxins are cleansed from the body.

Blue Vervain:

Blue vervain is recognized in Europe and elsewhere for its ability to reduce inflammation and fight fevers. It also helps to reduce muscle spasms. Blue vervain promotes perspiration adding to the cleansing action of white willow.

Feverfew:

Feverfew, as its name indicates, has been used for hundreds of years to reduce fevers. While it was undergoing a scientific study to confirm this action, it was noted that some of the subjects found relief from migraine. It has since been clinically studied for migraine and shown to be very effective especially in chronic conditions and in cases where other medications have failed. No one fully understands its method of action, but feverfew has been used for inflammation, asthma, and many other conditions with remarkable success. It is believed that feverfew works on migraines by reducing inflammation in the areas where pain is generated. Feverfew has gained broad acceptance in Britain, Canada, Israel and many other countries. Studies support whole leaf use rather than an extract.

Rosemary Leaves:

Rosemary performs two major functions in this formula: it relieves painful spasms and assists in reducing pain associated with rheumatism. Rosemary also improves liver function, promotes bile production, and assists digestion.

Skullcap:

Skullcap has gained recognition in many parts of the world. Its two main functions are the alleviation of nervous tension and sedation. Tension headaches, or headaches caused by lack of sleep, are often helped by skullcap. Skullcap is said to nourish the nerves.

Kelp:

Kelp's storehouse of micronutrients assist in many metabolic processes in the body. Kelp provides electrolytes which can help prevent edema. Edema and inflammation can be associated with conditions of excess fluid build-up, either in specific areas or generally throughout the body. Pain and inflammation are less likely to occur when the body's fluids are properly maintained. Kelp also contains algin which is mildly laxative and soothing to the gastrointestinal tract.

Other Supportive Nutrients

chamomile, lavender, bupleurum (chai hu), mistletoe, vitamin A, vitamin B-complex, calcium, iron, magnesium, potassium, zinc, omega-3 fatty acids, dl-phenylalanine, acidophilus

11

BLOOD HEALTH

FORMULA A:
BLOOD PURIFICATION

Indications:	Various viral and microbial infections, acn gout, and environmental toxin exposure
Recommended Formula:	Dandelion root, yellow dock, sarsaparilla roo burdock root, echinacea root, licorice roo cayenne, kelp
Dosage:	Four to six capsules daily. This formula shoul not be used for prolonged periods of tim greater than three months without a rest fror the formula for at least one month.
Contraindications:	High blood pressure
Doctor's Review:	Blood carries nourishment and oxygen to all th tissues, regulates the body's temperature an pH, and transports hormones to tissues wher they are needed. It also carries carbon dioxid and waste material away from the tissues to b filtered out and discharged from the body. It easy to understand why the health of the bloo is so important. Hypertoxicity of the blood ca occur when the liver is not functionin properly; the lungs are not transmitting enoug oxygen to the blood; when a person i overexposed to toxins through food medications, or environment; or when bloo fails to properly maintain pH or discharg waste. The health of the blood is greatl

influenced by the lungs, liver, lymphatic system and the kidneys. This herb formula will support each of these important systems of the body.

DOCTOR'S NOTES

Dandelion Root: A better tonic than dandelion, perhaps, has yet to be discovered. Dandelion supports the body's ability to detoxify by increasing perspiration, promoting urination, stimulating bile production and flow and improving liver function and bowel movement. It is reportedly able to cleanse and strengthen blood vessels. This common yard weed is officially recognized in France, Germany and Britain for its therapeutic benefits.

Yellow Dock: Yellow dock has some similar properties to dandelion root in that it promotes bile production and flow, has a mild laxative effect and works as a general tonic. It also helps with different skin diseases. This is probably why it is reported to be an excellent blood purifier and alterative. Many people believe that yellow dock is a rich source of iron, probably because it turns a rusty color as it matures. But a person would need to consume very large amounts of yellow dock (which is not recommended) to reach the U.S. recommended daily allowance for iron. Having said that, perhaps the iron that does exist in yellow dock is a highly absorbable form, so much less than RDA levels may be adequate. This area deserves more research. Yellow dock has been official in the *National Formulary* of the United States and is currently monographed in the *British Herbal Pharmacopeia*.

Sarsaparilla: Sarsaparilla has been used by many different cultures to treat a broad range of problems from arthritis to wounds. Its greatest reputation comes from its detoxifying and cleansing properties. Diuretic and diaphoretic effects are partly responsible for this reputation. Sarsaparilla's mild carminative action gives aid to those suffering from dyspepsia (indigestion).

Burdock Root:

Burdock stimulates and supports the body's detoxifying systems by serving as a mild laxative, diuretic, cholagogue (promotes bile production and secretion), and diaphoretic (promotes perspiration). The *British Herbal Pharmacopeia* makes note of its ability to detoxify. Germany, France and Belgium likewise recognize burdock root's cleansing applications.

Echinacea Root:

Some have referred to echinacea as the "king of blood purifiers." Healthy blood relies on the proper function of various organs. Echinacea helps maintain a healthy lymphatic system, and this results in cleaner, healthier blood. Echinacea also stimulates the production of white blood cells which helps to destroy invading toxicants. Discovered through its use by Native Americans it now enjoys recognition in Britain and Germany.

Licorice Root:

Licorice supports toxin removal by improving kidney and gastrointestinal tract function. Licorice is a mild laxative and diuretic. Its demulcent properties are soothing to the GI tract. Licorice is recognized throughout the world, but officially monographed in Britain, France, Germany, Switzerland, Belgium and Russia. However, its largest medicinal consumption is found in China.

Cayenne:

Cayenne is the herb in this formula that gets all going. Cayenne improves circulation which causes more blood to pass through the body's filtration system. For example, increased circulation causes more blood to circulate in the glomeruli of the kidneys and consequently more fluids are released as urine. Cayenne makes the other herbs of this formula more effective.

Kelp:

Kelp serves as an excellent source of trace elements which are cofactors in many and various metabolic processes. Without the presence of these trace elements, imbalances as well as organ and system dysfunctions can occur. This may ultimately result in less than healthy blood and body function. Kelp also provides soothing algin to the gastrointestinal tract which aids in keeping it healthier.

Other Supportive Nutrients

milk thistle, dong quai, poke root, sandalwood, pau d'arco, chaparral, red clover tops, carotene, vitamin C, vitamin E, niacin, glutathione, digestive enzymes

FORMULA B:
POOR CIRCULATION

Indications:	Poor circulation, phlebitis, cold extremitie varicose veins, and diabetes
Recommended Formula:	Cayenne, butcher's broom, kelp, gentian roo ginger, blue vervain
Dosage:	Two to six capsules daily. This formula may k used every day to help maintain health circulation.
Contraindications:	None
Doctor's Review:	Circulation of the blood is vital to the body. provides nutrients and oxygen to each cel Hormones are transported by the blood to tl tissues where they are needed. Blood carrie toxins and carbon dioxide away from the tissu to be filtered out and disposed of. When tl blood is not able to circulate properly, mild life-threatening conditions can occur. Som people may only experience cold hands an feet, while others may be subject t amputation, blindness, or even deatl Circulation can be impeded by various facto including plaque deposits in the arterie abnormal clotting and platelet aggregatio cardiac dysfunction or failure, and conditions shock. This herbal formula works to impro circulation.

DOCTOR'S NOTES

Cayenne:	Cayenne is perhaps nature's most perfe stimulating tonic. Cayenne stimulat circulation which improves the delivery nutrients and oxygen to cells, and discharg wastes and carbon dioxide from the bod Cayenne is particularly noted for improvir peripheral circulation. However, it can also he

stop and prevent external and internal hemorrhaging. Cayenne stimulates digestion and improves it, in part, by increasing saliva production. It increases perspiration which cleanses toxins from the blood. Cayenne reportedly has the capacity to prevent strokes and abnormal formation of blood clots. Since cayenne is a reputed pain reliever, it may have particular application for problematic circulatory pain, like that produced by phlebitis or thrombophlebitis. Considering its anti-spasmodic effect cayenne may improve conditions associated with Raynaud's syndrome.

utcher's Broom:

Butcher's broom has various effects on circulation. To illustrate, several thousand patients in France who were scheduled for surgery were given either a placebo or butcher's broom. About 36 percent of the patients on placebo developed unwanted and, in many cases, life-threatening blood clots. Less than two percent of the group on butcher's broom had clotting problems. This indicates that butcher's broom may have circulatory benefits for those going "under the knife ." There may also be applications for people in professions prone to injuries such as athletics. Butcher's broom shrinks blood vessels particularly in the legs. This helps to prevent that heavy feeling in the legs that some people, usually women, experience. In these people blood tends to pool up in the legs. Butcher's broom shrinks the vessels and pushes the blood back into the upper part of the body improving circulation throughout.

Kelp:

Kelp has a reputation of cleansing the blood vessels and preventing atherosclerosis. In those people who are iodine deficient, kelp can increase the metabolic rate which indirectly affects circulation in a positive way. Kelp

contains algin which is soothing to the GI tra
and mildly laxative. Kelp also contains tra
elements necessary for many metabol
processes.

Gentian Root:

Gentian has been used in folk remedies to tre
blood disorders. Gentian's real forte in th
formula is the ability to stimulate and impro
digestion. It also helps maintain a healthy liv
and spleen which effects both the blood ar
digestion.

Ginger Root:

Ginger root is noted for its carminativ
digestive, and circulation stimulating effec
Through its digestive effects ginger helps
liberate the active principles of the other herl
and through its circulatory effects ging
hastens the delivery of the actives to the sit
where they are needed. Sometimes improper
digested food components may be absorbe
into the blood which may trigger the bod
defenses. This could cause allergy symptom
Ginger improves digestion which may ke
unwanted compounds from being absorbe
into the bloodstream.

Blue Vervain:

Blue vervain is a time-tested favorite of mar
herbalists. It has had wide use in folk remedi
in Mexico, Brazil, and China. Blue verva
helps the blood properly clot when an inju
occurs and helps to keep blood vessels mo
pliable. It promotes mild perspiration, wat
loss, and bowel action, all of which help
maintain healthier circulation.

Other Supportive Nutrients

bilberry, gotu kola, ginkgo biloba, garli
vitamin B-6, vitamin C, niacin, omega-3 fat
acids, lecithin, l-carnitine, bromelain, fiber

12

CONSTIPATION

dications:	Constipation and when a soft stool is desired.
commended Formula:	Butternut root bark, cascara sagrada, senna leaves, ginger root, burdock root, Irish moss.
osage:	One to three capsules daily. Should not be consumed for more than seven days at a time.
ntraindications:	Pregnancy, lactation, and intestinal obstruction
octor's Review:	One of the largest health problems in the western world is in the area of elimination. Perhaps if the human family understood the full consequences that poor elimination has to health, then the knowledge to prevent many diseases would exist. While constipation does not directly cause one to miss many days of work or to be bedridden, it nevertheless causes a feeling of malaise or a sense of compromised health. Whenever the body cannot properly eliminate waste, which is full of toxic substances, many other of its systems become overworked and consequently perform at a compromised level, even shutting down altogether. Disease may progress more easily when the systems of the body are under stressful conditions.

The best solution for long-term control of constipation is diet. If meats are consumed they should be eaten in moderation. Adding more fiber-rich grams to the diet through whole grains, vegetables, and fruits will assist in returning elimination back to a healthy normal state. Some people believe that poor elimination is synonymous with poor diet.

Chronic constipation, in most people, is result of many years of a chronically poor diet. This herbal formula has a great laxative effec without the severe gripping caused by othe laxatives. This is also the best laxative formul to use when trying to restore normal bowe function. In addition to this, it is also ideal fo those individuals who experience constipatio only occasionally. However, keep in mind tha for most people, long-term control can only b achieved by diet modification.

DOCTOR'S NOTES

Butternut Root Bark:

Butternut does not cause all the gripping an discomfort associated with most laxatives. Thi makes butternut the laxative of choice for mos conditions. Most other laxatives, with long term use, will cause the body to becom dependent on them—but not butternut. I fact, combining butternut with other laxative such as the ones in this formula reduces th likelihood of the body developing a laxativ dependence. Therefore, butternut is ideal fo chronic constipation. The description o butternut's laxative effect as "soothing an tonifying" is well justified.

Cascara Sagrada Bark:

Cascara sagrada bark is an old Indian remedy Its name in Spanish means "sacred skin" o "sacred bark." Cascara is best when combinec with other herbs. Its laxative effect improve when the bark is allowed to cure for one to thre years before using. Cascara sagrada has beer listed in the *United States Pharmacopeia*, anc even though cascara is native to North anc South America, its reputation has given it officia recognition in Belgium, France, Germany Britain, and in other regions of the world.

Senna Leaves:

World-renowned senna is probably the mos widely used stimulant laxative even whe compared to synthetic drugs. Senna has undesirable side effects such as nausea and gripping that are alleviated when combined with other herbs, especially aromatics such as ginger. Like cascara, senna is officially recognized in many leading European countries.

Ginger Root:

Ginger root is the catalyst which turns what would otherwise be an ordinary laxative formula into the best formula available anywhere. While ginger root is not a laxative per se, it increases peristalsis by toning the intestinal muscle. However, its greatest achievements are probably found in its ability to improve digestion and prevent nausea, gas, and bloating. Since senna leaves can cause nausea and are best when combined with an aromatic herb, there is no better choice than ginger root. Ginger root's ability to fight nausea is well documented with one study published in the *Lancet,* showing it to be more effective than prescription motion sickness medications containing dimenhydrinate. Ginger also assists digestion through the action of its endogenous enzymes and second by stimulating bile flow.

Burdock Root:

Burdock root is an extremely mild laxative and an effective diuretic. It helps cleanse the body of accumulated toxins as a result of constipation. Its cleansing effect goes beyond its diuretic and laxative properties. It also promotes perspiration and strengthens the liver.

Irish Moss:

Irish moss has been used for centuries by people wanting to overcome intestinal problems. Irish moss contains high levels of mucilage which imparts a demulcent or soothing effect on the intestinal tract. It is also a nourishing food.

Other Supportive Nutrients

Yellow dock root, gentian, aloe resin, folic acid, acidophilus, bifidus, fiber

1 3

LIVER DYSFUNCTIONS

Indications:	Dysfunctional liver, hepatitis, jaundice, alcol cirrhosis, sluggish bile flow, gallstones, psoria:
Prescription:	Dandelion root, milk thistle seeds, burd root, peppermint leaves, artichoke, kelp
Dosage:	Two to four capsules daily. For chro conditions it is best to use maximum dosage four capsules per day for a prolonged period two to three months or until symptoms gone. May be used every day.
Contraindications:	None
Doctor's Review:	The liver is the largest organ and one of most vital to the body. Its functions inclu producing bile, processing and dischargi toxins and waste products, manufacturi energy-producing glucose from fats and ot substances, storing glycogen for quick ener regulating blood clotting, fighting disease, a maintaining of the body's hormonal balan These extensive functions clearly demonstr why the liver is so indispensable. It should just as clear that when the liver is unhealthy otherwise impaired, the ramifications to body can be enormous.

Just as there are many functions performed the liver there are   also many causes of li disease. Liver function can be disrupted bacterial and viral infections, overexposure toxic substances, excessive alcohol consum ion, obstruction of bile ducts, and by ot influences.

This herb formula is one of the best for treating various liver conditions. Whether the impairment is due to hepatitis, cirrhosis, toxins or obstruction, this formula can help. This is the only traditional herbal formula to incorporate dandelion, milk thistle, artichoke and peppermint—a very powerful and effective combination. Improvement in liver function is often noted by the amelioration of other conditions such as psoriasis.

DCTOR'S NOTES

ndelion Root:

Most people know from personal experience that dandelion roots penetrate deep into the ground. Dandelions use as a liver tonic is also deeply rooted. Dandelion has been used to treat liver and gallbladder obstructions, improve overall liver function, and promote bile production. Dandelion is a mild laxative and diuretic. Clinical use of dandelion is officially recognized in Britain, France, and Germany.

ilk Thistle:

Milk thistle is found in nearly every hospital emergency care and poison control center in Europe. It is used to protect the liver in cases of poisoning. Its liver protecting capacity is so remarkable that some of the most potent hepatotoxic substances known, such as those found in the "deathcap" mushroom, have a reduced impact on the liver protected by milk thistle. Normally, death would occur in a matter of hours after such a poisoning. Milk thistle increases production and storage of glutathione peroxidase in the liver. Glutathione peroxidase is a powerful antioxidant which provides protection to tissues of the liver and assists the liver in neutralizing toxins. Milk thistle also aids the liver in regenerating healthy tissue to replace damaged or diseased portions of the liver. A better liver tonic cannot be found anywhere.

Burdock Root: Burdock root promotes bile production an
                               secretion, but perhaps its best contribution
                               this formula is its ability to promo
                               perspiration, thereby reducing the load on t
                               liver to process and neutralize toxins. Oth
                               cleansing properties of burdock include its mi
                               laxative and diuretic properties. It has also bee
                               suggested in the treatment of gallstones.

Peppermint Leaves: Peppermint leaves are indicated whe
                               conditions of dyspepsia and sluggish bile flo
                               are encountered. However, peppermint al
                               supports the other herbs of this formula l
                               stimulating circulation and acting as a cataly
                               to increase overall effectiveness. Its carminitu
                               and anti-gas properties help it to countera
                               some of the GI tract irritation caused l
                               dandelion, milk thistle, and burdock. The
                               properties of peppermint have been time test
                               and demonstrated all over the world.

Artichoke: Although commonly recognized as a table foo
                               artichoke has been used historically to tre
                               various conditions such as jaundice, dyspeps
                               and decreased liver function. It supports b
                               secretion and acts as a mild diuretic.

Kelp: While it has been reported that kelp can he
                               with gallstones, its primary function in t
                               formula is to provide a rich supply of tra
                               nutrients as well as algin which is soothing a
                               mildly laxative to the GI tract.

Other Supportive Nutrients
                               turmeric, artichoke, vitamin B-12, vitamin
                               vitamin E, folic acid, lecithin, taurine, catechi
                               digestive enzymes, fiber

14

NERVOUS TENSION

Indications: Anxiety, nervous tension, emotional distress, restlessness, fear, hysteria

Recommended Formula: Valerian root, passion flower, wood betony, ginger, hops, skullcap, chamomile, blessed thistle

Dosage: Four to eight capsules daily

Contraindications: Low blood pressure

Doctor's Review: There are many situations, both emotional and physical, which contribute to anxiety. Many people are intimately aware of the things that cause stress and try whenever possible to avoid them. However, when stress becomes chronic, it may ultimately become the cause of many mild to serious physical disorders: difficulty in breathing, headaches, back and neck tension, and muscle spasms. If relief is not found for the aforementioned problems, immune function may become impaired which may eventually lead to greater illness or disease.

Since taking medication will not alleviate the causes of anxiety, the treatment of it must focus on symptom reduction. By treating the symptoms of stress, a person will better be able to relax, be calm, and even sleep well. This will help the individual cope with the underlying causes of the anxiety, while keeping the body in a better, uncompromised state of health.

Nature has provided botanicals comprising some of the best nervines, calming agents, and

relaxants known to mankind with very little
no side effects. These herbs have expertly be
brought together in this formula which w
help treat everything from tension and spas
to insomnia and digestive disorders.

DOCTOR'S NOTES

Valerian:

If this blend has a strong unpleasant odor, the
is nothing wrong. The odor is characteristic
valerian root. While the scent is hard to igno
the anxiety and nervous tension sufferer w
easily be able to look past it when valeria
effects are felt. Valerian is probably the m
widely used botanical in Europe for nervo
tension, anxiety and insomnia. In fact, the he
is found in dozens of drugs and te
Interestingly, valerian is calming and relaxing
cases of nervous tension and anxiety, while
the same time improving alertness and ability
concentrate. However, in cases of insomnia
will be more sedative. But note that consumi
too much valerian when fatigued can actua
be stimulating. Valerian seems to be just t
prescription for the modern human fami
considering its unusual versatility. As
interesting side note, valerian has also met wi
exceptional success with animals. Some ra
horses, become over anxious and nervous befc
a race. Many trainers have noted improv
performance after valerian root removed t
nervous edge.

Passion Flower:

Considering its name it might be misconstru
as the perfect aphrodisiac. However, befo
misconceptions arise, see Chapter 17 for t
origin of the name Passion flower. Passic
flower works well in formulas designed to tre
insomnia, but it works even better in formul
designed to combat stress, nervous tensio
anxiety, restlessness, hysteria and nervo

headaches. Passion flower promotes mild perspiration activating part of the body's cleansing and detoxifying system. Passion flower is officially recognized in many European countries including Britain, Belgium, France and Germany.

Wood Betony:

Wood betony has been well appreciated and prescribed for hundreds of years by old and new world physicians for treating nervous and sleep disorders, with particular application for tension headaches. It is a cleansing tonic to the blood and certain organs of the body. Along with valerian, wood betony is mildly carminative or in other words settling to the GI tract. Wood betony is officially recognized in the *British Herbal Pharmacopeia.*

Ginger Root:

Eating disorders and digestive disturbances often accompany nervous tension and anxiety. A better herb than ginger cannot be found to treat digestive disorders. Ginger assists almost every aspect of digestion. It stimulates saliva and bile production; prevents nausea, gas and bloating; improves peristalsis by toning the intestinal muscle; and optimizes friendly intestinal flora. Its ability to stimulate circulation makes the other herbs of this formula more effective. Ginger root activates the body's cleansing and detoxifying systems through its diuretic, diaphoretic (promotes perspiration) and digestive properties. Ginger root's therapeutic value is officially recognized in Britain, Belgium, and France.

Hops:

Hops is widely cultivated in North and South America, England, Germany and Australia for use in beer production. It has been so used for over a thousand years. Perhaps for just as long, hops has been used medicinally to treat restlessness, anxiety and sleep disorders. It is

prescribed for adults and children alike.
supports ginger root to help dispel flatulen
and ameliorate intestinal cramping. Ho
cleansrs and detoxifies through its diuret
effect. Hops is officially recognized in Britai
Belgium, France and Germany.

Skullcap:

Skullcap has proven itself useful for sle
disorders, nervous conditions, tremors, a
spasms. In earlier years it enjoyed offici
recognition in the *United States Pharmacope*
and the *National Formulary.* Skullcap is st
officially recognized in Europe to treat epilep
hysteria, nervous tension and insomnia.

Chamomile:

While chamomile has been modestly employ
in this country as a tea and in other heal
preparations, it does not even approach tl
success found in western and eastern Europ
especially Germany, where it is considered to
a panacea or cure-all. Chamomile has be
extensively researched where it has demonstrat
usefulness in sleep and digestive disorders. It
carminative or settling to the GI tract, but a
mildly stimulating to the bowel without being
true laxative. It is officially recognized in Britai
Belgium, France, and Germany.

Blessed Thistle:

Blessed thistle plays a supporting role in tl
formula. It helps activate a sluggish liver a
correct stomach and digestive problem
flatulence and tension headaches. It furth
supports the body's cleansing and detoxifyi
systems by promoting perspiration ar
removing excess fluids. Britain, Germany ar
Belgium officially recognize its medicinal valu

Other Supportive Nutrients

lavender, lady slipper, kava, ginkgo bilob
catnip, vitamin B-complex, vitamin C, calciu
magnesium, unsaturated fatty acids

15

LOW ENERGY

Indications: Fatigue, chronic low energy, weakness, low stamina

Recommended formula: Cayenne, Siberian ginseng, gotu kola, kelp, peppermint leaves, ginger root

Dosage: Four to six capsules daily. May be used for up to three months at a time.

Contraindications: None

Doctor's Review: Fatigue, chronic low energy, and weakness have become common place in modern society. These conditions can be caused simply by a lack of rest or excessive activity, in which case the solutions may be elementary. However, if the condition is caused by other factors such as malnutrition, circulatory problems, heart disease, anemia, respiratory problems, infectious diseases (especially those where toxic substances are produced), endocrine disturbances, anxiety, etc., then the solution may be much more challenging.

This herbal formula is designed to help in overcoming many of the above listed obstacles, but without the use of harsh or unhealthy stimulants like caffeine. For example, Siberian ginseng helps to combat both mental and physical stress, and cayenne, ginger and peppermint aid digestion and improve nutrition. It is easy to overuse or abuse stimulants, but this formula is hard to abuse. Nevertheless, a few weeks' break should be taken periodically.

DOCTOR'S NOTES

Cayenne:

Cayenne is perhaps nature's best stimulating tonic. It improves digestion, circulation, and toxin removal from the body. Cayenne will help if weakness and chronic fatigue are due to malnutrition as a result of a poor digestion. It will also assist if weakness and chronic fatigue are caused by poor circulation which can prevent vital nutrients and oxygen from getting to the various cells of the body and waste products from being removed. If weakness and chronic fatigue are caused by toxins in the blood then cayenne, with its ability to promote perspiration and stimulate urine production can be of use.

Siberian Ginseng:

Siberian ginseng is very effective in combating mental and physical stress. It is interesting to note that while using ginseng people working rotating shifts will adapt to a new schedule more rapidly. Also, people using ginseng can handle larger work loads and are better able to withstand adverse conditions. Russian athletes have discovered that ginseng enhances their performance. Mental stressors such as neurosis, anxiety, and hyperchondriasis are helped with ginseng. Ginseng increases a sense of well-being. It also reduces high blood pressure and arthrosclerotic conditions. Ginseng is simply one of the best multi-directional stimulating tonics available.

Gotu Kola:

Gotu kola's main application in this formula is its circulation stimulating effect and its ability to treat nervous system disorders. Also, evidence suggests that it may destroy harmful toxin producing bacteria. In addition to this, gotu kola is a mild diuretic which can help maintain a cleaner system. It has been considered a longevity promoting herb, but this use has not been substantiated. Nevertheless, it is a wonderful tonic herb and an effective addition to this formula.

elp:

Kelp contains many trace elements, the most notable being iodine. Iodine deficiency can cause hypothyroidism which leads to lethargy, obesity, and general malaise. Kelp also contains a soluble fiber called algin which is soothing to the GI tract and improves bowel function. Kelp's other trace elements can assist in various metabolic processes in the body.

eppermint Leaves:

Peppermint is, of course, a common flavoring agent, but it also has been used for thousands of years for medicinal purposes and as a stimulant. Peppermint is used throughout Europe to improve digestion and reduce gas, nausea, and nervous headache. It quiets spasms and helps with insomnia. It improves breathing which will make more oxygen available for the body.

inger Root:

Ginger, like peppermint, is a wonderful carminative herb and exhibits many of the same effects. It reduces spasms, improves digestion, increases circulation (especially peripheral circulation), improves bowel function and reduces inflammation. It is officially recognized in Britain, Belgium and Germany.

ther Supportive Nutrients

astragalus, damiana, elecampane, angelica, panax ginseng, valerian root, vitamin B-complex, vitamin C, iron, magnesium, manganese, potassium, zinc, l-aspartic acid, l-carnitine, coenzyme Q10, inosine, octacosanol, fiber

16

PROSTATE TROUBLES

Indications:
Enlarged prostate (benign prostat
hypertrophy, BPH), prostatitis, frequency
urination

Recommended Formula:
Saw palmetto berries, pumpkin seeds, cornsi
parsley leaves, ginger root, nettle root, kel
burdock root

Dosage:
Four to eight capsules daily. For chron
conditions it is best to use maximum dosage
eight capsules per day for a prolonged period
several months or until symptoms subside. M:
be used on a continuous basis.

Contraindications:
As with any diuretic product potassiu
supplementation may be necessary to preve
potassium depletion if used in large amoun
for an extended period of time.

Doctor's Review:
Prostate problems whether mild or severe affe
50 percent of the male population over the a
of 45. Some experts believe that if all men liv
long enough, 100 percent of them would suff
prostate problems. For men, prostate cancer is
leading cause of death. This formula does n
have the ability to cure prostate cance
However, when used prophylactically th
formula does have the ability to help maintain
healthy prostate gland. And a healthy prosta
gland is less likely to degenerate into a disease
state. So it is conceivable that by using th
product regularly, even in the absence
prostate problems, some of the more serio
diseases, possibly including cancer, might b

avoided. Nevertheless, the more serious applications for this product include enlarged or inflamed prostate conditions.

Several of the herbs (or their constituents) of this blend have been the subject of a number of clinical studies for the treatment of prostatic enlargement. Side effects caused by the most popular prescription drug product makes this formula an attractive alternative, as it is more effective and virtually free of side effects when used as directed. As a word of caution, most men suffering prostate problems have nothing more than enlargement and inflammation, but symptoms can be the same as those experienced by the few men that suffer prostate cancer. Prostate cancer, when caught early, is one of the most treatable forms of cancer so be sure to have a proper diagnosis by medical professionals.

DOCTOR'S NOTES

Saw Palmetto Berries:

Clinically, saw palmetto berries have a rich history of use beginning earlier this century with the natural doctors. Saw palmetto berries gained official recognition in the *National Formulary* and today a specialized extract of the berry has become the product of choice for enlarged prostate conditions in many European countries, including Germany. The United States Food and Drug Administration, as recorded in the *Federal Register,* has acknowledged that saw palmetto effectively reduces symptoms associated with enlarged prostate conditions. Scientific research has demonstrated that saw palmetto is an effective *5-alpha reductase* inhibitor which essentially means that the male hormone, testosterone, will be kept in a form that does not cause prostate stimulation. Saw palmetto also inhibits the production of leucotrienes which are compounds in the body associated with the inflammatory processes. These berries have a mild diuretic affect. This is a tremendously useful herb for the modern maturing man.

Pumpkin Seeds: Pumpkin seeds have been used for centuries as a diuretic and to treat urinary tract disorders. In recent years a clinical trial was performed in Sweden, demonstrating that the oil fractions of pumpkin seeds and saw palmetto berries, when combined, made an effective prostate enlargement remedy.

Cornsilk: Cornsilk has received official recognition as a diuretic in the United States as well as Europe and is found in many traditional European diuretic formulas. Cornsilk contains high levels of mucilage which provides a soothing or demulcent effect for the urinary and GI tracts.

Parsley Leaves: Parsley is a well known diuretic receiving official recognition in France, Germany, and Britain. Apiole, a constituent of parsley, has an ability to keep spasms in check, which may assist with spasms that occur in the pelvic region of those suffering prostatic enlargement.

Ginger Root: Ginger is a spice known throughout the world but most people are unaware of the research, both chemically and clinically, that has been performed on ginger. For example, ginger is known for its anti-inflammatory properties. This may be explained by the fact that research has demonstrated that ginger has an ability to inhibit prostaglandin production in the body. Some prostaglandins are involved with the body's inflammatory processes. Ginger also has the ability to keep spasms in check. Ginger contributes to this formula in several other ways. It promotes perspiration which helps to cleanse the body. Its also settling to the GI tract and stimulating to the circulatory system.

Nettle Root:	In one clinical study, nettle root was shown to be very effective in reducing prostatic symptoms. Even with long term use of over four years nettle root exhibited an ability to maintain a healthy prostate.
Kelp:	Kelp contains a storehouse of trace elements, including iodine, for which it is well known. Kelp has been used for many different conditions but is of special note for this formula because of its historical applications for the male genitourinary tract. It also provides mucilage to gently cleanse and soothe the GI tract.
Burdock Root:	Burdock root provides overall support to the other herbs of this formula helping to make them better able to perform their function. Burdock root also promotes perspiration and acts as a diuretic. In addition to this, it has received a reputation as a blood purifier.

Other Supportive Nutrients

cranberry, prickly pear flower, *Pygeum africanum*, flower pollen extract, goldenseal root, kava, vitamin B-6, selenium, zinc, essential fatty acids, l-alanine, l-glutamic, l-glycine, oligomeric proanthocyanidins, phytosterols

17

INSOMNIA

Indications: Insomnia, nervous sleep disorders

Recommended Formula: valerian root, hops, skullcap, passion flower, dandelion root, chamomile, marshmallow root, hawthorn berries

Dosage: Two to four capsules daily

Contraindications: Should not be used when driving or operating heavy equipment or with conditions of low blood pressure.

Doctor's Review: Insomnia is a condition that afflicts many people. Its root causes are many and diverse. The two primary causes, however, are anxiety and pain. In other words insomnia is not the problem, but simply a symptom of the problem. Nevertheless, if insomnia is not corrected it can cause development of other illnesses or conditions. Even the immune system can be compromised by insufficient rest and sleep. In acute conditions, natural pain medications and sleep aids can be useful and quite often necessary. For chronic conditions, sufferers should eliminate the underlying cause. This herbal formula can treat symptoms associated with anxiety and mild pain, but sedation is its real forte.

DOCTOR'S NOTES

Valerian Root: Valerian root's volatile oil produces a strong unpleasant odor. Some people jest that even if valerian had no sedative therapeutic quality, the odor alone is enough to knock a person out

However, valerian does have significant therapeutic value as demonstrated by the many scientific, clinical and pharmacological studies as performed to date. More importantly is the fact that millions of people all over the world can attest to valerian's sedating effects. There are literally dozens of pharmaceutical and tea preparations throughout Europe which employ valerian's tranquilizing benefits. One should not confuse valerian with the popular drug valium as they are not related in any way. Valerian is officially recognized in Britain, Belgium, France, Germany, Switzerland and Russia.

Hops:

If the name "hops" rings a bell it is probably because you have heard it associated with beer production. In fact, hops has been used for over a thousand years to produce beer. Less commonly known, and dating back to early times, is hops' medicinal use. Hops has a sedative effect which has been well documented. Even the people collecting hops for beer production have been known to become abnormally sleepy while working. Hops has a calming effect on the nervous system which helps with insomnia and restlessness, particularly that associated with anxiety. Hops also provides a cleansing action related to its diuretic properties. Britain, Germany, France, and Belgium all officially recognize the medicinal value of hops.

Skullcap:

Skullcap brings even more sedative action to this herbal formula. This plant has proven itself useful for sleep disorders, nervous conditions, tremors, and spasms. Skullcap supports the body's waste removal system by its diuretic and diaphoretic actions. Skullcap is officially recognized in Europe. Its uses there include sedation, as well as for epilepsy, hysteria, and nervous tension. Skullcap was official in the *United States Pharmacopeia* from 1863-1916, and in the *National Formulary* until 1947.

Passion Flower:

The name passion flower originated back in the late 1500s and early 1600s. Apparently it physical attributes reminded someone symbolically of the things associated with the week of Christ's passion or crucifixion, and therefore has become known as "passion flower." Note that its consumption has not been shown to engender passion. It is widely used in Europe as a sedative and to treat common nervous conditions including nervous headaches and restlessness. It is officially recognized in Britain, Belgium, France and Germany and has been listed in the *National Formulary* of the United States.

Dandelion Root:

Dandelion root plays a supportive role in this formula, even though it has no sedative or anti anxiety action. It does have a mild laxative effect which helps cleanse the body and return it to a more normal state of health. Quite often conditions of anxiety and pain cause digestive disorders. Dandelion root helps to improve the digestive system by stimulating bile production and flow. Dandelion root is considered to be a good tonic in support of general well being. It is officially recognized in Britain, France, and Germany.

Chamomile:

In Germany, chamomile is considered to be a panacea, or cure-all. Its main use throughout Europe, however, is associated with its ability to help with digestive and mild sleep disorders. It has been the subject of a tremendous amount of chemical, scientific, and pharmacological research. At a recent international scientific conference held in Germany, approximately 10-15 percent of the scientific presentations were surrounding the study of the constituents and benefits of chamomile. Chamomile supports the overall sedative properties of this formula and provides a carminative action which is settling to the gastrointestinal tract. Chamomile is officially recognized in Britain, Belgium, France and Germany. It also has wide use here in the United States as a tea.

Marshmallow:

Marshmallow is accepted in Britain, Belgium, France, and Germany as an emollient and demulcent. Its demulcent properties provide soothing activity for the gastrointestinal tract, improving digestion. Marshmallow root does not have any sedative action, but plays a supporting role in this herbal formula.

Hawthorn Berries:

Hawthorn's cardiotonic benefits are well documented in Europe. Hawthorn has an ability to dilate blood vessels, particularly the coronary vessels which increase blood flow to the heart and reduce overall blood pressure. It will also help to tonify the heart muscle, which is beneficial in situations where the heart muscle itself has been damaged, or the effects of aging are felt. Indirectly, these heart related benefits provided by hawthorn may help but they do not fully justify hawthorn's inclusion in this calming or sedating herbal formula. While its cardiotonic benefits may improve overall feeling of well-being it has two lesser known properties. Hawthorn berries have been used as a mild tranquilizer as well as an antispasmodic. Interestingly, hawthorn berries have been incorporated in many European natural sedative formulas.

Other Supportive Nutrients

American ginseng, kava, schizandra berry, lavender, vitamin C, vitamin E, inositol, niacinamide, calcium, magnesium, melatonin, Chinese herbal combination called suanzaorentang

18

OBESITY

Indications:	Obesity, excess weight
Recommended formula:	Chickweed, celery seeds, psyllium seeds, horsetail, fennel seeds, Irish moss, kelp, white willow
Dosage:	Six to ten capsules daily. Should be used daily.
Contraindications:	None

Doctor's Review:

Obesity is a common problem which is directly or indirectly responsible for many other health problems. Obesity has no single underlying cause. Sometimes it can be the result of disorders which are associated with psychogenic, genetic, thyroid and hypothalamic problems that can be complex and difficult to diagnose. Essentially the underlying cause creates a condition where more energy is consumed in the form of food than the body burns. The excess energy is converted to fat and stored in the body. Since obesity is a complex condition, a herbal formula designed to address several of the more common underlying causes is most appropriate. This herbal formula is excellent in treating various primary and secondary causes of obesity. Any weight loss effort should include consulting a health care professional, exercise, and fat and calorie control for maximum and lasting benefits.

DOCTOR'S NOTES

Chickweed:

Chickweed is considered by many herbalists to be one of the better appetite suppressant herbs.

Its weight control applications, however, do not stop here. Chickweed cleanses plaque from blood vessels and is able to break down and eliminate fatty substances from the body. Many people who are subject to food cravings and addictions find that cleansing fasts (which should be done only under the direction of a health care professional) can eliminate cravings and specific food addictions. It is believed that a cleansing fast removes compounds from the body that cause the cravings. Once the cravings are gone it is advisable not to consume the food that was formerly craved, as it may trigger more cravings. Chickweed supports the cleansing action by stimulating the body s own system of elimination. Chickweed is diuretic, mildly laxative and a soothing demulcent to the GI tract.

Celery Seeds:

Celery seeds provide stimulation and tone to the body. This helps return the body to a positive energy state. In other words, the amount of energy consumed is equal to the amount of energy burned. Less energy will be converted to fat. Celery also prevents muscle spasm so exercise to your heart's content. Celery is an excellent diuretic and diaphoretic (promotes perspiration). This property will be of use in cleansing the body of toxins whether or not one chooses to fast. Many herbalists have used celery to help those people with a tendency for obesity.

Psyllium Seeds:

Psyllium seeds provide a bulking, water soluble fiber which promotes bowel elimination and cleansing. Psyllium will absorb many times its weight in fluids causing appetite cessation while contributing very little in calories. Psyllium, like other fibers, has an ability to reduce serum cholesterol and remove fatty substances from the body. Scientific studies have demonstrated psyllium's usefulness in weight control.

Horsetail (Shave Grass):   Horsetail is a mild diuretic and has traditionally been used in Europe as an adjuvant in weight loss diets. It stimulates the body's metabolism. In addition to this, horsetail contains silica which is essential in maintaining a stronger healthier skeleton, which can be beneficial to obese and overweight people whose skeletons are often in a stressful and sometimes compromised state. Horsetail is used and officially recognized in Belgium, France, Britain, and Germany.

Fennel Seeds: Fennel seeds, like several other herbs of the formula, are mildly diuretic. Fennel has a strong carminative action which reduces flatulence and bloating. Like celery, fennel reduces spasm and may prove useful during and after exercise. Fennel helps the bowel to better adapt to the laxative effect produced by some of the other herbs.

Irish Moss: Irish moss is an excellent mucilage containing demulcent. The mucilage is similar to psyllium in that it absorbs large amounts of fluids and imparts a feeling of fullness. In this way it is an appetite suppressant. Irish moss is considered to be very nutritive. Overweight people quite often have nutrient imbalances that can be helped and possibly fully corrected by Irish moss.

Kelp: Obesity is quite often associated with the dysfunction of thyroid gland. Kelp, like Irish moss, is very nutritious. However, kelp's iodine content also helps to maintain normal function in the thyroid gland which is the main reason for its addition to this formula. The thyroid gland regulates metabolism and controls the use of oxygen and heart rate. Kelp contains algin which is another soluble fiber and further adds mucilage and bulking to this formula.

White Willow: White willow does not seem to have any direct applications for weight loss or obesity but still has been included in several traditional weight loss formulas. White willow has been used for thousands of years as a pain medication. Obese and overweight people are often prone to more aches and pains than others. This can occur partly because they are probably out of shape and partly because the excess weight adds more stress to the joints increases the likelihood of pain. Certainly when an out-of-shape person starts an exercise regimen, muscle soreness and tenderness will abound.

Other Supportive Nutrients

ginseng, garcinia cambogia, burdock root, vitamin B-complex, vitamin C, vitamin E, calcium, chromium, magnesium, phosphorus, unsaturated fatty acids, lecithin, l-carnitine, l-glutathione, coenzyme Q10, fiber

19

GLANDULAR AND CENTRAL NERVOUS SYSTEM TONIC

Indications: Nervous and glandular weakness and disorders

Recommended Formula: Goldenseal root, gentian, Siberian ginsen
                                chamomile, blue vervain, dandelion roo
                                yellow dock root, skullcap, wood betony, kel
                                ginger root, saw palmetto berries

Dosage: Two to four capsules daily

Contraindications: None

Doctor's Review: There are various glands in the body whic
                                perform a variety of functions. The purpose
                                the body's many glands is to secrete substanc
                                that are necessary for life, physical and ment
                                health, and normal bodily functions. Son
                                glands may secrete a single substance whi
                                others may secrete several substances
                                complex mixtures. The glands secrete suc
                                things as digestive enzymes and bile, hormone
                                saliva, perspiration, and mother's milk. It is ea
                                to understand why glandular health is vita
                                However, in order to have good glandul:
                                health it is necessary to have a healthy nervo
                                system. It is the nervous system th:
                                orchestrates glandular secretions, and when tl
                                glands and nervous systems are in good healt
                                the body works like a well directed orchestr
                                This formula contains herbs that will tonify ar
                                nourish both the glands and the nervous system
                                It can correct imbalances and improve health.

Goldenseal Root:

Goldenseal root is considered to be one of the best tonics. Its applications are not strictly confined to glandular and nervous system support. However, goldenseal can treat liver problems and improve bile production and secretion. It will also improve genitourinary function. A unique property of goldenseal is its ability to fight bacterial infections. Some glands such as the prostate gland are subject to a higher incidence of infections that may be helped by goldenseal root. Goldenseal will improve the central nervous system and produce a mild sedative effect. Goldenseal's mild laxative effect will stimulate internal cleansing and improve overall health.

Gentian:

Gentian is considered by most Europeans to be the best herbal digestive tonic. Gentian improves digestion right from the beginning of the digestive process by increasing the secretion of saliva. It has further been demonstrated to increase bile production and secretion. Its digestive benefits are officially recognized in Britain, Germany, France and Switzerland. Some herbalists have used it wherever general debility exists.

Siberian Ginseng:

Siberian ginseng is considered to be an *adaptogen* which is a substance that normalizes function irrespective of the direction of dysfunction. This is very important to glandular and nervous system function since both the glands and nervous systems can be hypoactive or hyperactive. Siberian ginseng has a protective effect on the adrenal and thyroid glands by preventing atrophy (wasting) caused by cortisone, thyroidin, and other compounds. Siberian ginseng has a clinically supported reputation as a stress fighter. It helps the body to cope with stress and maintain proper

function when subjected to stressfu
environments. Stress can over excite the nervou:
system and induce glandular dysfunction sucl
as in the cases of thymic and lymphati
involution (reduction in size and power).

Siberian ginseng has been used to increase
reproduction capacity and sperm counts ir
animals. Siberian ginseng also provides :
protective effect against radiation exposure
Siberian ginseng improves internal cleansing
ability by helping renal function and increasing
renal capacity.

Chamomile: Chamomile is held in high regard in Germany
                          where it is considered to be a panacea or cure
                          all. Its main applications in this formula are
                          related to its nerve tonic and relaxing
                          properties, and its ability to improve digestion
                          Chamomile has a profound ability to calm the
                          nerves and reduce tension. Chamomile i
                          popular and officially recognized in Britain
                          France, Belgium, and Germany. Even in the
                          United States it is used as a bedtime tea.

Blue Vervain: Blue vervain is a favorite tonic of many
                          herbalists. It assists in disorders of the splee
                          and liver. When the liver is dysfunctional, :
                          greater stress is placed on the other cleansing
                          and eliminating mechanisms of the body. Blu
                          vervain stimulates perspiration to help the
                          body's internal environment. Blue vervain ca
                          break the cycle in recurring nervous problems
                          Although its effect is mild, it has beer
                          considered a natural tranquilizer.

Dandelion Root: Dandelion root is another favorite of many
                          herbalists as a tonic with particular application
                          for the liver. It improves liver health and bil
                          production. It is said to be able to cur
                          obstructions from the gallbladder and spleen
                          Dandelion's cleansing benefits are due to it

diuretic and mild laxative effects. Dandelion is officially recognized for its medicinal value in Britain, France and Germany.

Yellow Dock Root:

Yellow dock root has very similar uses and applications as dandelion root. Yellow dock supports bile production, improves digestion, treats spleen and lymphatic disorders, and improves skin health. Some people believe yellow dock's iron component may be more absorbable which can assist with production of hemoglobin.

Skullcap:

Skullcap was once found in the pages of the *United States Pharmacopeia* and the *National Formulary* for its tranquilizing and anti-spasmodic properties. It is still officially recognized in Europe where it is used to treat nervous tension, hysteria, and epilepsy.

Wood Betony:

Wood betony has been used for hundreds of years by natural healers to treat various nervous disorders. It is still used to treat anxiety, tension headache and hysteria. It is also used to treat nerve inflammation and faulty nerve nutrition. It assists in reducing the effects of nerve toxins.

Kelp:

Kelp contains many trace elements that assist in various metabolic processes in the body. Possibly none is more important than iodine, which helps to maintain proper thyroid function. In Japan where significant amounts of kelp are consumed, there is a lower rate of many diseases including breast cancer, obesity and thyroid problems. Potassium, magnesium, sodium, and other important trace elements found in kelp, are nerve nutrients. Kelp contains algin which improves bowel function and soothes the GI tract.

Ginger Root:

Ginger root supports the digestive and elimination systems of the body through its

carminative and perspiration-promotin
properties. Ginger root further exhibi
antispasm and anti-inflammatory propertie
Perhaps its most important contribution to th
formula is its ability to enhance the actions o
the other herbs and improve circulation.

Saw Palmetto Berries: Clinical studies have demonstrated sa
palmetto berries' effect in treatment of enlarge
prostate in men and difficult menstruation an
pelvic congestion in women. It seems to exert
hormone balancing effect irrespective of gende
Saw palmetto berries were used by Nativ
Americans in Georgia and Florida for th
treatment of urinary disorders.

Other Supportive Nutrients

milk thistle, lady slipper, gotu kola, ginkg
biloba, valerian root, multiple vitamin
multiple minerals, evening primrose oi
coenzyme Q10, fiber

20

GASTROINTESTINAL TRACT

lications:	ulcers, flatulence, upset stomach, diverticulitis, gastritis, colic, irritable bowel syndrome, most GI tract disorders.
:ommended formula:	goldenseal root, licorice root, papaya leaves, gentian root, myrrh gum, Irish moss, fenugreek seeds, ginger root, aloe vera gel
sage:	Two to four capsules daily
ntraindications:	None
ctor's Review:	Gastrointestinal problems are common and for the most part can be avoided with the proper diet which means moderate meat intake and sufficient fiber. Two much meat increases bowel transit time and fails to properly clean the GI tract. Too little fiber can lead to constipation, diverticulitis and other GI tract disorders. Recent serendipitous discoveries have shown that some peptic ulcers are caused by a particular bacteria. Several herbs in this formula also have a positive effect in the treatment of ulcers. Nausea and flatulence are common GI tract problems that many people would like to avoid. This formula contains herbs that will treat the most common of these disorders and help treat the symptoms of some GI tract disorders that are genetically inherited.

CTOR'S NOTES

denseal Root:	Goldenseal root is native to North America where it has been used by Native Americans as a powerful tonic. Today it is popular for many

applications with credit being given to the r
alkaloid content. Goldenseal root is antise
and may show positive activity against the u
causing bacteria called *H. pylori.* Goldenseal
been used to restore the mucus lining of the
tract and keep it from being easily disrupted
strengthening the cross linking of protein
the mucus. Goldenseal promotes bile secret
restores proper bowel transit time and rem
excess water from the body. Goldenseal h
positive influence on most of the common
tract problems.

Licorice Root:

Licorice root has been medicinally used for
3,000 years. Many of its actions are simila
those of goldenseal root. Licorice has b
clinically researched for its ability to t
gastric ulcers. Approximately 37 percent of
ulcers disappear and many others are reduce
a consequence of licorice use. A constituen
licorice known as *glycyrrhizin* has sho
promise against bacterial and viral activ
Perhaps its anti-ulcer activity is due at leas
part to this antiseptic property. Still m
believe that the anti-ulcer activity is relate
its ability to stimulate the gastric mucos
secrete more mucus. Licorice is furt
recognized for its anti-inflammatory acti
which can help in cases of gastritis. Licorice
a diuretic and mild laxative effect that clea
toxins from the body. Licorice is u
medicinally by the people of western
eastern Europe and is widely used by
Chinese. The licorice in this formula is
licorice, which is not used in most lico
candies in the United States. True licoric
used in some European candies.

Papaya Leaves:

Both papaya fruit and leaves are a sourc
papain which is a mixture of protein diges
enzymes. Carbohydrate- and fat-digest
enzymes are found to a much lesser deg

With this understanding it is no surprise that papaya leaves are used to assist digestion in cases of dyspepsia. They have also been used to expel intestinal worms.

ntian Root: Gentian enjoys widespread use particularly in Europe as a digestive aid. It increases saliva and is believed to increase secretion of gastric juices. Some herbalists have used it to expel intestinal worms. It benefits conditions of heartburn and indigestion, and its anti-inflammatory effects are helpful with gastritis. It is considered a bitter tonic.

yrrh Gum: Myrrh gum has been medicinally used throughout the world. It has been used for almost every type of common bacterial infection, thus it may have an effect against the ulcer-causing *H. pylori* bacteria. Myrrh gum is used to heal the gastric mucosa which may further help with ulcers. Myrrh gum is carminative, reducing gas and bloating, and calming the stomach. It also is a mild laxative.

sh Moss: Irish moss is rich in trace mineral nutrients. It also contains large amounts of mucilage which soothes the GI tract. It is specifically used for dyspepsia, nausea, and heartburn. Some herbalists suggest Irish moss for diarrhea.

nugreek Seeds: As much as 40 percent of the weight of fenugreek seeds is mucilage. Mucilage is a gelatin-like substance usually made up of proteins and polysaccharides. Most consumable herbal products that contain high amounts of mucilage have been employed for stomach and intestinal ailments. Fenugreek seeds are no different and have been administered for these very purposes.

nger Root: Ginger is one of the best herbs for the treatment of digestive disorders. Ginger prevents nausea, gas, bloating, and vomiting Ginger is particularly beneficial in cases c pancreatic dysfunction. One study published i the British medical journal *Lancet* prove ginger to be more effective for motion sicknes than the prescription medication containin dimenhydrinate. Ginger root is not a laxative but it will tonify the intestinal muscle.

Aloe Vera Gel:

Aloe vera gel is a clear jelly-like material calle mucilage. Aloe has been successfully employe in treating irritable bowel syndrome. Aloe g improves bowel transit time, reducin putrefaction in the intestinal tract, and increase friendly bacteria like acidophilus.

Other Supportive Nutrients

angelica, catnip, vitamin A, vitamin B-complex vitamin C, vitamin E, multiple minerals acidophilus, bifidus, digestive enzymes glycosaminoglycans, water, formula describe in chapter 27

21

INFECTIONS

Indications:	General and chronic infections, fever, cold, flu, sore throat
Recommended Formula:	Echinacea, goldenseal root, myrrh gum, garlic, licorice root, blue vervain, butternut root bark, kelp
Dosage:	Six to twelve capsules daily. Should not be used for more than three weeks at a time.
Contraindications:	None
Doctor's Review:	It may be true that a cure for the common cold has yet to be discovered, but until that discovery is made there are some promising herbs that are quite effective at reducing the symptoms and duration of colds, flu, and infections. At the top of the list is echinacea, goldenseal, myrrh gum and garlic. This herbal formula includes these four ingredients and is designed to fight viral and bacterial infections, enhance and support immune response, reduce fevers, cleanse the body and improve health. This formula is not just for those suffering colds and flu, but it is for infections of varying types and origins.

DOCTOR'S NOTES

Echinacea:	Some herbs and other products have been called "cure-alls," but very few have lived up to the title. Echinacea root, however, is about as close as anything that comes to a cure-all. Echinacea is native to North America and has been used by Native Americans to treat snake

and insect bites, and infections. Tod:
echinacea is becoming one of the mc
recognized herbs in the world for its medici
value. A tremendous amount of scienti:
documentation is mounting supporting
various uses. In the United Kingdom it is us
to fight chronic, viral and bacterial infectio:
pathogenic organisms in the blood, boi
various skin complaints, colds and influenza.
Germany it is used to treat infections of t
head, nose and throat.

Echinacea has met with great success in treati
wound infections and ulcers. Recently certa
peptic-ulcers were shown to be caused by
bacteria called *H. pylori*. It is possible th
echinacea exerts bactericidal effect against t
organism or perhaps stimulates the immu
response to better control it.

Immune stimulation is another well know
property of echinacea. It stimulates t
ingestion and digestion of foreign bacteria a:
matter by immune system cells call
phagocytes. It also improves mobility
infection combating leucocytes (white bloc
cells). Some studies indicate that echinacea c
stimulate *interferon* which is a protein th
protects cells from viral attack.

Some people ask which species of echinacea
best—*purpurea* or *angustifolia?* However,
doesn't really matter which one is used as th
seem comparable in function and ability. As
point of caution, some herbs like *Partheni*
integrifolium have been substituted for the tr
echinacea and labeled as echinacea. Do:
accept substitutes and insist on the real plant.

Goldenseal Root: Goldenseal root, considered by the Cherok
Indians to be a powerful tonic, is still used
many people today. Many of the more sensiti

and infection-susceptible tissues of the body are protected by a mucus lining. This mucus lining helps to keep out viruses and bacteria. When the mucus lining is weak or disrupted, pathogens can more easily enter and cause infection. Goldenseal root is recognized by many herbalists and natural healers as possessing an ability to strengthen the mucus lining, making it harder for pathogens to penetrate. Two of goldenseal's more active compounds, hydrastine and berberine, have demonstrated effectiveness in treating ulcers and various bacterial and viral infections, especially those of the respiratory tract. Goldenseal's assistance in this formula continues as it also acts as a mild diuretic and laxative which cleanses the body and provides an internal environment more conducive to optimal health.

rrh Gum: Myrrh gum has some similar properties as found in echinacea and goldenseal root. Myrrh gum stimulates phagocyte activity and reduces inflammation of the mucus secreting mucosa. Myrrh gum also helps with skin problems, ulcers, and acts as an antiseptic and anti-inflammatory. Myrrh gum is officially recognized in Britain, France, and Germany for its medicinal value.

lic: Garlic is another herb that can be considered a tonic. It is a powerful warrior against infections of various types and origins but is particularly applicable to GI tract infections and disorders. It is used to treat dysentery and just about any intestinal infection. Because garlic stimulates bile flow, it has shown promise with conditions such as irritable bowel syndrome which can actually be a side effect of dysentery. Cholera and typhoid are other infections that garlic can be helpful in treating. Garlic helps to expel intestinal worms. Also, candida yeast infections respond moderately to garlic therapy. Garlic c increase the number of leucocytes (white blo cells) which help fight infections. In additio garlic increases perspiration which furth cleanses the body. Garlic is considered to be carminative which improves digestion a reduces gas and bloating.

Licorice Root:

Licorice root contributes in several importa ways to this formula. It stimulates secretion the hormone aldosterone from the adren cortex. This can produce a higher energy lev which is usually needed when combatir infections like colds.

Licorice has antiviral and antibacterial activi which may help with *H. pylori*-induced ulce Licorice is also considered a demulcent which soothing to the GI tract. The demulcent effe is due to its ability to stimulate gastric muco which increases mucus secretion. This is t most commonly cited reason for its anti-ulc activity. In addition, licorice root is a gen laxative which contributes to internal cleansir Long-term consumption of licorice is n recommended as it may cause weaknes electrolyte imbalances, water retention a hypertension. Licorice is officially recogniz for therapeutic activity in Britain, Franc Germany, Belgium, China and many oth countries.

Blue Vervain:

Blue vervain has an ability to expel intestir worms and break the cycle of chronical occurring infections. It has been used for col and flu and has an ability to reduce fever.

Butternut Root Bark:

Butternut is a laxative that is used to tre dysentery and diarrhea. It also has an ability expel worms. While it is a laxative, it does r produce the sometimes painful grippi associated with other laxatives. Butterno improves liver function and stimulates bile production and flow.

lp:

Kelp's function in this formula is to provide needed trace elements important in many metabolic processes in the body. These nutrients may further support the healing process and return the body to normal function. Kelp contains a soluble fiber called *algin* which is soothing to the GI tract and improves bowel function.

ther Supportive Nutrients

astragalus, cranberry, elderberry leaf and berry, isatis (ban lan gen), propolis, St. John's wort, pau d'arco, vitamin A, vitamin B-complex, vitamin C, vitamin E, iron, magnesium, phosphorus, selenium, zinc, essential fatty acids, acidophilus, dimethylglycine, grapefruit seed extract

22

COUGHS AND SORE THROAT

Indications:	Colds, sore throat, bronchial congestion an inflammation, coughs
Recommended Formula:	Bayberry root bark, horehound, ginger roo slippery elm bark, cloves, cayenne
Dosage:	Six to twelve capsules daily. May be taken a long as condition persists.
Contraindications:	None
Doctor's Review:	The common cold is the number one reaso people miss work and school. As colds ar highly contagious it may be best for people t stay at home and recuperate which requires be rest and relaxation. Colds that are accompanie by regular or constant coughing, hacking an congestion can be some of the most difficult t overcome since they often do not allow fo sufficient rest. Those conditions may als interfere with the proper rest and relaxation o others living in the same dwelling. This formul contains the best herbs known for reducin coughs, bronchial congestion and spasms, an sore throats.

DOCTOR'S NOTES

Bayberry Root Bark:	Bayberry root bark has been used for centurie and is considered by some herbalists to be on of the most valuable medicinal herbs Apparently others held bayberry in high regar since it was official in the *National Formular* until 1936. Bayberry helps increase secretion o mucus which can soothe dry sore throats. It ha

also demonstrated an antiseptic effect against various pathogenic organisms. Bayberry relaxes and opens bronchial tubes for easier breathing. Bayberry stimulates bile flow improving digestion. It is considered to be a very nutritious herb which combined with its circulation stimulating action quickly gets nutrients to the tissues that need them most. Bayberry modestly increases perspiration which cleanses the body of unwanted toxins.

Horehound:

Many people will recognize the name horehound from its use in horehound candy. Horehound has been used since ancient times to treat coughs, colds, sore throats, and bronchitis. It is very beneficial as an expectorant, removing phlegm from bronchial cavities. Horehound has received particular praise for treating chest colds and reducing hard, hacking, painful coughs. It also treats other respiratory ailments such as hoarseness and asthma, and reduces bronchial spasms. In addition, horehound improves bile flow and functions as a mild laxative. Its internal cleansing action includes a diuretic and perspiration promoting effect.

Ginger Root:

Ginger root is probably the best digestive and carminative herb employed today. It improves circulation, especially in the periphery. Its circulatory and digestive action improves the effectiveness of the other herbs. Ginger stimulates saliva production which can be helpful with dry coughs. Ginger exerts an anti-inflammatory action in bronchitis. It also works to cleanse the bowel and promote perspiration.

Slippery Elm Bark:

Slippery elm bark has a remarkably high mucilage content with exceptional nutritional value. It is easily digested and used as a food in convalescence. The mucilage is soothing to the GI tract and improves digestion. Slippery elm is

antitussive (anti-cough) and anti-inflammato
It works to soothe raw sore throats.

Cloves: Cloves are another excellent carminativ
aromatic herb with many properties like tho
of ginger root. Cloves are a very mild pa
reliever taken internally but are much mo
powerful when applied directly. Sore throa
may benefit from this action. Cloves furth
assist coughs that are accompanied by bronchi
phlegm. Cloves' antiseptic and disinfecta
properties may treat underlying infections.

Cayenne: Cayenne has been employed by herbalists ar
natural healers around the world to treat col
and their symptoms. It is, perhap
understandable that something with so mu
heat is used to treat a condition called "a cold
Cayenne is used to break up congestion, redu
chills, and improve bronchial conditions ar
sore throats. Like the other carminative herbs
this formula, cayenne stimulates digestion ar
circulation. With improved circulation mo
urine is usually produced which may provide
healthier internal environment.

Other Supportive Nutrients
echinacea, isatis (ban lan gen), St. John's wo
licorice, vitamin A, vitamin B-complex, vitam
C, vitamin D, vitamin E, zinc, unsaturat
fatty acids, bioflavonoids, water, formu
described in chapter 21

2 3
EYE DISORDERS

Indications: Eye infection, conjunctivitis, dry eyes, inflamed eyes, eye strain

Recommended Formula: Eyebright, goldenseal root, red raspberry leaves, dandelion root, fennel seeds, slippery elm bark

Dosage: Four capsules daily. May be used regularly.

Contraindications: Avoid applying directly to the eyes.

Doctor's Review: Surely the eyes have fascinated humanity since prehistoric times. They have been called the windows to the soul. Iridology has been used by various cultures and natural healers for thousands of years as a diagnostic tool for detecting ailments. Most people take the miracle of eyesight for granted. It seems the eyes are subject to an ever increasing bombardment of abuse. With the advent of computer monitors, eye strain is much more common today than in past decades. Environmental pollutants, stress, injury, and nutrition have a profound effect on the health of the eyes. An appreciation of eyesight is quickly gained when a person has to do without it, even if only for a short time. This herbal formula serves as an eye tonic to promote good eye health and reduce the discomfort associated with various ocular disorders including infections.

Doctor's Notes

Eyebright: In a nutshell the name of the herb speaks for itself. The name "eyebright" comes from the flower's appearance which reminds the beholder of a bright open eye. A number of therapeutic agents have been discovered based on the appearance of a botanical resembling the thing it is treating. Eyebright is a good example and so is ginkgo biloba. Ginkgo biloba leaves are shaped like the hemisphere of the brain. Today hundreds of studies have demonstrated ginkgo's positive effect on the brain. This is called the doctrine of signatures.

Eyebright has been found to be useful in a number of different eye disorders including eye strain, bloodshot eyes, conjunctivitis, irritations, and dry or weeping eyes. Eyebright is also noted for its astringent qualities. Astringents are agents that shrink tissues and blood vessels. This may help in treating bloodshot eyes to reduce the unpleasant cosmetic and physical effects especially in chronic conditions. Eyebright has never been studied scientifically to try to substantiate these uses. Nevertheless, personal testimonials and anecdotal evidence abound. Its use dates back thousands of years and today enjoys official recognition in the *British Herbal Pharmacopeia* where it is indicated for, among other things, conjunctivitis. It also suggests that it be used in conjunction with goldenseal root which is discussed in the next paragraph.

Goldenseal Root:

Goldenseal root is considered to be a powerful tonic herb. Its two primary benefits for the eyes are found in its ability to fight infections and improve the health of mucus membranes.

Conjunctivitis is a condition of inflammation of the mucus membranes located on the inside of the eyelids (the conjunctiva). Conjunctivitis is often caused by invading pathogenic organisms. Goldenseal root has a long history of use in improving mucosal health throughout the body. Unhealthy conjunctiva can lead to sore, dry, itchy eyes and, in more extreme cases, blindness. Goldenseal provides secondary benefits by improving digestion and stimulating and cleansing the bowels.

ed Raspberry Leaves: Red raspberry leaves have astringent qualities which may be used to reduce the size of vessels in bloodshot eyes especially if conditions are chronic. Red raspberry leaves are soothing and healing to mucus membranes such as those found on the inside of the eyelids. Red raspberry has been used by Native Americans in treating sore and inflamed eyes. It is officially recognized in Britain for its therapeutic value in treating conjunctivitis.

andelion Root: Dandelion root has many indirect actions that can improve the health and appearance of the eyes. Dandelion stimulates the body's various cleansing and waste removal systems. It is mildly laxative and improves bowel function, stimulates urine flow, and promotes mild perspiration. Dandelion is an excellent liver tonic and improves digestion by causing an increase in bile secretion. By improving liver health, conditions of jaundice can be overcome such as yellowing of the white portion of the eyes.

nnel Seeds: Fennel seeds are used to impart a licorice scent to candies and have been used in food for perhaps thousands of years. Its medicinal applications relate to digestive disorders including gas, bloating and colic.

Perhaps its main application in this formula is to improve digestion and the effectiveness of the other herbs. Still it has been found beneficial in treating eye inflammation, conjunctivitis and blepharitis (inflammation of the edge of the eyelid).

Slippery Elm Bark:

Slippery elm bark contains copious amounts o very nutritious mucilage. It has been used as food in convalescence. It is soothing, demulce and mildly laxative to the GI tract. Slippery e benefits many mucus membranes including t conjunctiva.

Other Supportive Nutrients

bilberry, ginkgo biloba, butcher's broo vitamin A, beta carotene, vitamin B-comple vitamin C, vitamin D, vitamin E, calciu chromium, magnesium, phosphorus, seleniu zinc, glutathione, taurine, lutein, quercetin

24
PARASITES

Indications:	Parasites and worms
Recommended Formula:	Garlic, black walnut hull, butternut root bark, myrrh gum, Irish moss
Dosage:	Four to eight capsules daily. Treatment should stop only after the parasites or worms have been fully removed from the body and proper bowel function is restored.
Contraindications:	None
Doctor's Review:	A parasite is an organism that lives off another organism (the host) to the detriment of the host. If the host is a human, there is no such thing as a friendly parasite. Parasites come in different sizes and shapes and cause a variety of problems, many of which can be life threatening. Some worms and protozoa are types of parasites. Parasites can enter the host through the mouth, insect bites, or skin.

The best therapy for parasites is prevention. Quite often an infection can be prevented through proper hygiene, by using insect repellents, and precautionary procedures like boiling untreated drinking water. The best treatments are those that quickly expel the parasite with the least impact on the host. The aftermath of a parasitic infection can leave the body in disrepair like a forsaken battleground. The intestinal tract may remain dysfunctional for some time, during which cramping, spastic or otherwise irritable bowel symptoms can abound.

This formula treats the problems and consequences of parasite infections. It contains herbs that have been used to treat parasite infections safely for centuries. It is particularly beneficial in treating intestinal parasites but can have a strong, destructive effect on parasites found in other regions of the body. This formula is also great to use as a preventive measure when there is a risk of parasite infection.

DOCTOR'S NOTES

Garlic:

Garlic has been used for centuries to treat viral, bacterial, and parasitic infections. Its applications for parasites include worms and protozoa in the intestinal tract and elsewhere in the body. Because some of the parasites that garlic is effective against are able to leach the blood, it may be from this that the myth about vampires and garlic's ability to ward them off was generated. Garlic conditions the GI tract and returns it to a state of health once an intestinal parasite infection is cleared. Garlic possesses the ability to prevent infection especially if it is one that is contracted through insect bites. When garlic is consumed in sufficient quantities (a gram per day), its odor can be detected through the pores of the skin creating a natural insect repellent.

Black Walnut Hull:

Black walnut hulls have been nearly as popular as garlic over the years in treating parasite infections. Unlike the other major herbs of this formula, black walnut has an ability to kill the parasites while the other herbs expel them. It has also been found effective in treating ring worm and other types of fungal diseases.

Butternut Root Bark:

Diarrhea is a common problem in some parasite infections. Butternut root bark has been successfully employed to treat dysentery and diarrhea. It is reputed to be useful in treating fungal infections as well as tapeworms. Some have used it to treat syphilis. Butternut root bark has a laxative effect without causing diarrhea. It is one of the only laxatives to be free of gripping.

Myrrh Gum: Myrrh gum is used to treat various infections including those caused by parasites. Myrrh gum promotes the secretion of mucus keeping the protective barrier lining the intestines and other tissues in better condition and making it harder to disrupt. Thus, myrrh gum can help to prevent infections since some parasites, in order to infect, must disrupt the protective mucus barrier. Also increased mucus production has a restorative effect on GI tract function after the parasites are gone. Myrrh gum has demonstrated an ability to stimulate some of the body's immune responses.

Irish Moss: Irish moss provides a soothing mucilage to the GI tract. This mucilage has been used for years as a source of food in convalescence. Irish moss improves bowel function and prevents diarrhea.

Other Supportive Nutrients
artimisia annua, wormwood, vitamin A, vitamin B-complex, vitamin D, vitamin K, calcium, iron, potassium, unsaturated fatty acids, acidophilus, bifidus

25

ENVIRONMENTAL TOXINS

Indications:	Overexposure to environmental pollution, heavy metal toxicity, poor diet, accidental toxin consumption, recovery from illness
Recommended Formula:	Pectin, algin, psyllium husk, Irish moss, alfalfa leaves, kelp, myrrh gum
Dosage:	Four to six capsules daily. May be used on a continual basis.
Contraindications:	None
Doctor's Review:	The whole idea of cleansing any area of the internal body other than the colon is foreign to Western medicine. When a doctor thinks of internal cleansing, it is usually in the form of a laxative or colonic. However, many other cultures around the world recognize a more complete internal cleansing as a means to restore and maintain health. Quite often a more complete comprehensive cleansing includes fasting. Fasting helps the body rid itself of accumulated toxins whether they are from radiation, factory or auto emissions, or food. This formula contains herbs that cleanse, absorb and remove toxins from the body, increase resistance to damage from toxin exposure, and provide a rich source of nutrients that will nourish weakened tissues as a result of overexposure to toxins.

DOCTOR'S NOTES

Apple Pectin:	Apple pectin is the glue that holds the cells of the apple together. It performs the same

function in apples as collagen does in humans. Apple pectin is a soluble, indigestible fiber which has a pronounced effect on improving bowel function and health. Many toxins cleansed from the blood by the liver are secreted from the liver with the bile. As the bile enters the intestinal tract, the pectin binds to the toxins preventing their reabsorption into the bloodstream. They are then carried out of the body. Pectin has demonstrated an ability to lower cholesterol. Its mode of action remains a subject of debate. However, many speculate that it binds with cholesterol preventing its absorption into the blood.

Many toxins enter the body through foods. Fasting, or at least reducing the amount and types of foods consumed, can have a positive impact on internal cleansing and health. First, it gives the body's organs a chance to rest, recuperate, and heal. Second, it gives the body a chance to operate with minimal toxin exposure. Apple pectin, along with other soluble fibers found in this formula, helps to reduce food intake by giving the sensation of being full without adding calories. Pectin expands turning into a thick jelly-like substance as it absorbs many times its weight in fluids. It is this property that makes it so popular as a thickener in jams and jelly.

Algin:

Algin is very similar to pectin; however, algin is derived from a sea vegetable called kelp. The algin in this formula is separated from the kelp so that it is in a highly concentrated form. Algin is another soluble fiber which helps to remove toxins from the body especially heavy metals. It appears to have the ability to bind with bile salts, preventing dietary cholesterol from being absorbed. To the extent that algin bonds to toxins, it protects tissues of the body that would otherwise come in contact with the toxins and thus be damaged. It also improve the health of the good bacteria found in the G tract. Some people underestimate th importance of intestinal flora, which ca process and dispose of toxins. Also this health promoting flora keeps pathogenic micro organisms, many of which produce toxi chemicals, from becoming too numerous.

Psyllium Husk:

Psyllium husk is another botanical that i acclaimed for its soluble fiber. It too absorb toxins, improves bowel function by supplyin bulk, and increases good flora. Both psylliu seed and psyllium husk have large amounts c soluble fiber. Psyllium husk was chosen for th formula to limit overall caloric intake.

Irish Moss:

Irish moss adds yet another source of solubl fiber to this formula. It helps to cleanse th fluids of the body. Irish moss is used as an easil digested and nutritious food for convalescents.

Alfalfa Leaves:

Alfalfa is a nutrient-dense herb and has been staple in animal feed for many years. Ofte animals are fed a much more nutritious an healthy diet than people. Alfalfa is consumed b many people as a means of improving nutritio and it is consumed by others for cleansing an healing. Alfalfa is a herb that does not requi pesticides to grow, which is anothe consideration for people trying to remov toxins from the body and diet.

Kelp:

Kelp is in this formula as the concentrated algi all ready discussed and again as the whole se vegetable. It improves nutrition as a rich sourc of trace elements. Kelp is a great source c iodine which assists the thyroid gland in number of different metabolic processes. Als iodine protects the thyroid gland from radiatic exposure.

Myrrh Gum: Myrrh gum improves the mucosa which
                              provides a protective barrier to keep toxins from
                              penetrating the tissues. It is also recognized for
                              its ability to cleanse the GI tract. Myrrh gum is
                              a fighter of infection and can reduce toxins
                              produced by pathogenic organisms.

Other Supportive Nutrients
                              cloves, milk thistle, ginseng, myrrh gum,
                              oregano, rosemary, vitamin A, carotene, vitamin
                              C, vitamin E, selenium, glutathione, oligomeric
                              proanthocyanidins

26
THYROID DYSFUNCTION

Indications: Thyroid dysfunction, overweight, hypo-
                           thyroidism, hyperthyroidism, goiter

Recommended Formula: Kelp, Irish moss, Siberian ginseng, gentian root,
                           fenugreek seeds, cayenne

Dosage: Two to four capsules daily. May be used
                           continuously.

Contraindications: None

Doctor's Review: The health of the thyroid gland plays a
                           significant role in the quality of life. The
                           thyroid gland secretes various hormones, and a
                           dysfunctional gland can either secrete too much
                           (hyperthyroidism) or too little hormone
                           (hypothyroidism). If too much hormone is
                           secreted, a person can experience heart
                           palpitations, weight loss, nervousness, and
                           excessive sweating. If too little hormone is
                           secreted, a person may experience obesity,
                           reduced muscular activity, tiredness, general
                           malaise, low energy, and depression. Many
                           herbal products have been found that influence
                           thyroid function and health. Many of the mild
                           to moderate cases of dysfunction can be helped
                           simply by modifying the diet to obtain iodine
                           and other trace elements. This formula contains
                           herbs that provide iodine and have been
                           clinically proven to improve thyroid function.

DOCTOR'S NOTES

Kelp: Kelp contains many trace elements. The most
                           prominent and beneficial for thyroid function

is iodine. Iodine is essential to the thyroid gland and in the production of thyroid hormones. Iodine deficiency is known to produce obesity, goiter, dull, dry skin and hair, and a reduced basal metabolic rate. Iodine can also protect the thyroid gland from radiation toxicity. Kelp contains many other beneficial elements like algin, which soothes and cleanses the gastrointestinal tract.

Irish Moss:

Irish moss is a seaweed which, like kelp, contains iodine. The many benefits described in the previous paragraph on kelp also apply to Irish moss. Irish moss contains mucilage which is soothing to the GI tract.

Siberian Ginseng:

Siberian ginseng maintains a strong tonic effect on the entire body. This effect improves overall health and function of the body. Siberian ginseng has a specific and powerful influence on the thyroid gland. It protects the gland from enlargement induced by thyroidin and atrophy induced by methylthiouracil. Siberian ginseng has a clinically supported reputation as a stress fighter and energizer. Siberian ginseng also protects against radiation exposure. It is used throughout the world and officially as a medicine in France, Germany, and the United Kingdom.

Gentian Root:

Gentian root is a tonic which has been used for many years to treat most chronic diseases and general debility. Its main use in this formula is to improve digestion and strengthen the human constitution. It is widely used in Europe where it has found official recognition in France, Belgium, the United Kingdom, and Switzerland.

Fenugreek Seeds:

Fenugreek contains mucilage which improves bowel function. It is very nutritious and supplies needed nutrients throughout the body. Many herbalists consider it to be restorative, turning dysfunctional systems of the body to a state of good health.

Cayenne:

Cayenne makes the other herbs of this formula much more effective. It accomplishes this by stimulating digestion and improving circulation. Thus, it delivers actives and other micro-nutrients faster and with greater intensity to the thyroid gland. Cayenne is mildly diuretic which is a side benefit to its ability to stimulate circulation.

Other Supportive Nutrients

artichoke, damiana, vitamin B-complex, vitamin C, vitamin E, protein

27

DIGESTIVE DISORDERS

Indications:	dyspepsia (indigestion), colic, flatulence, heartburn, poor digestion, antibiotic therapy, pancreatic insufficiency, dependence on laxatives
Recommended Formula:	papaya leaves, peppermint leaves, fennel seeds, ginger root, gentian root, cayenne, Irish moss, butternut root bark
Dosage:	Two to three capsules daily. Best if taken during a meal.
Contraindications:	Should not be used when pregnant.
Doctor's Review:	Consumption of antibiotics, a dysfunctional liver and pancreas, old age, stress, and poor diet are major contributing factors to digestive health. Digestive disorders can lead to many illnesses and in advanced cases the illnesses can be quite serious. Chronic digestive problems are of the greatest concern since they usually cause the more serious illnesses.
	Even though digestion does not officially begin until food enters the mouth, the way the food is prepared can impact its digestibility. After chewing the food, the process of digestion continues until finally the waste is expelled from the body. Constipation is one of most common symptoms of digestive disorders.

This formula can free a person fro
dependence on laxatives. It contains herbs th
improve all digestive functions and work
many different ways. No prescription or ove
the-counter medicine will improve digestic
and then maintain function as well as th
herbal formula. This formula is ideal for peop
who have the ability to swallow capsules.

DOCTOR'S NOTES

Papaya Leaves:

Papaya leaves are a rich source of an enzyn
called papain. Papain is ideal for people wi
pancreatic insufficiency because it is a prote
digesting enzyme which functions in a simil
way to the body's own pepsin and pancreat
protease enzymes. Papain also contains sm;
amounts of lipase (fat digesting enzyme) ar
amylase (carbohydrate digesting enzyme
Papaya contains chlorophyll which is a
effective internal deodorizer. Disagreeable od
quite often accompanies digestive disorder
Papaya has also shown effectiveness in expellir
tapeworms.

Peppermint Leaves:

Peppermint leaves contribute to this formula
several ways. If nervous disorders are the cau
of poor digestion or vomiting, peppermi
helps by calming the nerves and relaxing th
muscles of the GI tract. Peppermint likewi
can help to calm a spastic intestine an
cramping stomach. Bile is an important fact
in healthy digestion and occasionally it
almost non-existent in some digestive disorder
Peppermint increases bile production an
secretion. It helps prevent heartburn, nause
gas, and colic. Peppermint also stimulates th
bodies elimination systems. Britain, Franc
Belgium, Germany, Switzerland, and Russia a
among the many countries that official

recognize and accept peppermint's remarkable influence on digestion.

nnel Seeds:

Fennel seeds have a wonderful aroma that many people associate with licorice. The aromatic oils are believed to be responsible for fennel's powerful effect on the digestive system. Fennel is calming to the stomach and soothes stressed spastic muscles of the GI tract. It can relieve colic and reduce flatulence. A common side effect to many digestive disorders is constipation. Fennel reduces the need for laxatives and prevents the gripping discomfort often associated with their use. Fennel's diuretic action further supports the cleansing and healing process.

inger Root:

There's probably not another herb that more fully supports the digestive process than ginger. It has been used for thousands of years by many cultures around the world. As an example, ginger is consumed heavily by the Japanese, especially with sushi. They use it to clean and freshen the pallet, stimulate saliva secretion, and improve digestion. A modern scientific study shows ginger to have a powerful ability to prevent motion sickness and is even more effective than prescription motion sickness medication. This demonstrates ginger's amazing carminative action in soothing and settling the stomach. Ginger improves circulation and transports nutrients to the cells that may be malnourished because of poor digestion. Ginger also normalizes the action of the intestinal muscle. Cleansing of the body is accomplished by ginger's diuretic effect.

ntian Root:

Gentian is a very popular European bitter used to treat and prevent digestive disorders. Applications for gentian include indigestion,

heartburn, vomiting, low bile and saliv
secretion, and dyspepsia. Gentian is officiall
recognized in Germany, France, Belgium an
the United Kingdom.

Cayenne:

Cayenne is a powerful stimulant to circulatio
and digestion. Since poor digestion can result i
malnutrition, improving digestion an
circulation together will speed the recover
process. Cayenne is used to treat gas, colic, an
GI tract spasms. Though some people may fin
it hard to imagine, cayenne has successfull
treated ulcers by deadening the exposed nerve
and preventing internal bleeding. It appear
that fighting fire with fire in some cases doe
indeed work.

Irish Moss:

Irish moss is employed in this formula for it
soothing demulcent properties. It contain
mucilage which coats the GI tract and improve
the integrity of the lining. It is this property fo
which Irish moss has successfully treate
gastritis and other GI tract disorders lik
diarrhea. Irish moss is also very nutritious an
found to be helpful in convalescence.

Butternut Root Bark:

Butternut root bark has a soothing laxativ
effect that does not cause gripping. Its use
include treatment of constipation, diarrhea
dysentery, and intestinal worms.

Other Supportive Nutrients

angelica, catnip, vitamin B-12, vitamin C, foli
acid, acidophilus, activated charcoal, catechin
digestive enzymes, formula described in chapte
20

28

HEALTH AND BODY TONIC

Indications: Stress, malaise, low energy, fatigue, body system imbalances, and general debilities

Recommended Formula: Sarsaparilla root, Siberian ginseng, astragalus, fo-ti, gotu kola, saw palmetto, licorice root, kelp, alfalfa, ginger root, stillingia

Dosage: Four to eight capsules daily. Can be used continuously as a general tonic.

Contraindications: None

Doctor's Review: Fatigue is one of the most common complaints people present to their primary care physician. Sometimes the cause of fatigue can be easily revealed through laboratory tests. Some causes are a low functioning thyroid, low levels of red blood cells (anemia), and candida yeast infections. However, it is not uncommon for people to undergo numerous lab tests which do not reveal the cause of their fatigue.

It is very likely that the underlying cause of fatigue is stress. Stress is responsible for numerous and varied health problems within individuals, based partly on their previous health history, genetics, and how they view the stress they are under. Because the causes of stress are varied and multiple, it is important that people who have an unknown cause of

fatigue visit their physician to obtain a base lin
laboratory test, so they can be sure that thei
stress is not caused by hypothyroidism, anemia
candida, or some of the other causes of fatigu
that can be determined by a blood test.

Nevertheless, the majority of people wit
fatigue illness have absolutely normal bloo
studies. Therefore, iron or thyroid therap
holds no promise for such people, an
alternative ways of treating this commo
complaint must be employed. This herba
formula is an invaluable tool in treating non
specific fatigue that may be caused b
underlying stress· or other undiagnosed factor
This formula is ideal as a general tonic as it ha
the ability to improve just about all aspects c
health.

DOCTOR'S NOTES

Sarsaparilla:

Sarsaparilla is an alterative. *Webster's Dictionar*
defines alterative as something that graduall
restores healthy body function. Sarsaparilla ha
been used as a food and medicine by Nativ
Americans. Rheumatism, gout, skin and live
disorders are among the conditions helped b
sarsaparilla. Native Americans used it to trea
general debilities. It is also known to contai
hormone precursors that are believed to hel
balance hormone function in both gender
Sarsaparilla was employed as a blood purifier i
the 1800s and today is well recognized for th
cleansing action caused by its diuretic, mil
laxative and perspiration promoting effects.
has gained official recognition in Germany an
the United Kingdom.

erian Ginseng: Siberian ginseng has a clinically demonstrated ability to block the effects of stress. Ginseng is also good for stimulating energy production in the body. Many nervous system disorders are effectively treated with Siberian ginseng. It has a tonic effect on the central nervous system.

tragalus: Astragalus is one of the most prominent herbs in all of Chinese medicine. The reason it is used so much is because it strengthens and readies the body's immune function. In other words, it helps the body fight and overcome a myriad of ailments and potential ailments by strengthening the immune system. Astragalus will not stimulate the immune system to action, but prepares it so when an immune response is required it functions at a higher level.

-Ti: Fo-ti contains very powerful antioxidants which can be useful in treating many common maladies including hypertension, high blood cholesterol, and weakness. Fo-ti has been used to promote longevity. This is because of reports of people living about 150 years and attributing this remarkable phenomena to the consistent use of fo-ti. The actual birth dates of these allegedly long-lived people were not able to be documented. Nevertheless, fo-ti improves kidney function and blood health, and contains anti-aging antioxidants which may actually contribute to a longer life.

tu Kola: Gotu kola has been used in ayurvedic medicine as a central nervous system tonic. Studies have shown it to improve mental function including memory and ability to learn. Gotu kola improves circulation which can help the body to recover more rapidly from various disorders.

It also is very useful in helping to maint
healthy skin and helping the skin to repair it
after injury. However, gotu kola is m
specifically an anti-fatigue herb.

Saw Palmetto Berries: For men, saw palmetto berry is most w
known for its ability to protect and maintai
healthy prostate. For women, it decrea
ovarian, uterine irritability and relieves pair
periods. It will help to normalize ovar
function. It appears to have a hormc
balancing effect for both genders.

Licorice Root: Licorice root's unique effects inclu
antibacterial and anti-viral properties. It a
affects estrogenic activity which can be help
in females, but is not harmful to males. Lico
root in any herbal formula helps to modul
and strengthen activity of other herbs that
present.

Kelp: Kelp is a plant from the sea. It contains ma
nutrients beneficial to the body's metabc
processes. Kelp has been shown in epidem
logical studies to decrease the incidence
breast cancer. It treats thyroid disea
hypertension and helps with arthritis. Kelp a
contains algin which is soothing to the GI tra

Alfalfa: Alfalfa, like kelp, is very nutritious and much
its benefit can be attributed to this property
can stimulate the appetite and has no equal :
spring tonic. It is beneficial in treating pain
chronic conditions like arthritis.

Ginger Root: Ginger root improves and maintains a heal
digestive system. Perhaps no other herb
such broad applications or performs as well

ginger. Ginger improves circulation and makes the other herbs of this formula more effective. Well known for its carminative action, ginger prevents gas and bloating.

llingia: Stillingia, like sarsaparilla, is described as an alterative which restores proper body function. Stillingia has been used in many ways to treat such diverse conditions as cancer and eczema.

ther Supportive Nutrients

sage, dong quai, reishi mushroom, shiitake mushroom, maitake mushroom, multiple vitamins, multiple minerals, unsaturated fatty acids, acidophilus, bifidus, fiber

29

DEGENERATIVE DISORDERS

Indications:	Cancer, Addison's Disease, rheumatism, ski disorders
Recommended Formula:	Red clover blossoms, licorice root, pau d'arc barberry root bark, stillingia, sarsaparilla roo prickly ash bark, cascara sagrada, burdock roo buckthorn bark, kelp
Dosage:	Six to eight capsules daily. May be used ever day for treatment and during convalescence.
Contraindications:	None
Doctor's Review:	Cancer is a degenerative condition that is a unfortunate fact of life for too many peopl Arguably, much of the cancer that plague society could be prevented with the prope lifestyle, diet, occupation, and environmen Even though cancer often seems to come o suddenly, the body may have been chronicall subjected to stressors that led to the cancer i the first place. While it is true that 100 percer of people with malignancy will not recover an indeed die of complications attributed to th cancer, others will completely recover with n apparent explanation even when the cancer ha progressed beyond the point of what seemed t be a rational hope of recovery. Perhaps peopl who would otherwise die recover when thei bodies are given a little of the right support.

In the early part of the 1900s, a man named Hoxsey had an herbal formula he claimed cured cancer. Many people that were cured of cancer while under his care agreed. Whether it was his formula that cured them or they were cured by unrelated reasons is still disputed to this day. Most of the major herbs of the Hoxsey formula are also found in this formula. In fact, Hoxsey combined 10 herbs and eight of them are found in this formula. These herbs may provide needed support to overcome cancer or other serious degenerative diseases. This formula also contains three ingredients not found in the Hoxsey formula that make it much better. A person may choose to use this formula as an adjunct to other therapies. Because of the serious nature of cancer, it is important that the individual explore all potential treatments and consult with a health care professional.

DOCTOR'S NOTES

Red Clover Blossoms:

Red clover has found its way into most herbal cancer treatments as a primary ingredient. However, red clover's use in treating cancer is not supported by scientific research. It has been used as an alterative. In fact, early naturopathic doctors found that it gradually restored overall health. Skin cancers may be prevented if the skin is better maintained and red clover blossoms, along with many other herbs in this formula, are particularly beneficial at maintaining healthy skin.

Licorice Root:

Licorice root is one of the herbs that is found in the Hoxsey formula. Its main purpose was to make the formula more palatable. However, Hoxsey may or may not have known that licorice also helps to modulate and strengthen activity of the other herbs. This property licorice's main function in this formu However, licorice does impart many otl qualities which prove very useful degenerative diseases. Many degenerati diseases and their treatments sap the ener from a person. Licorice increases adrenal gla function to stimulate energy. Licorice beneficial in the treatment of Addison's dise (a deterioration of the adrenal glands). Peo with degenerative diseases are usually fighti stress which is another condition helped licorice. Cleansing is also very important recovery from degenerative diseases. Licor supports the cleansing functions as a diure and a mild laxative. It is also soothing to the tract.

Pau d'Arco

Pau d'arco is a popular modern herbal can treatment. The therapeutic constituent cal *lapachol* has been shown in animal studies to very effective in treating various types of canc and tumors. In these studies, it had little or side effects when consumed in the whole pl form, but in a human study caused naus vomiting, and blood thinning when used in purified chemical form. This type of experie is understandable since mother nature oft combines, in the plant's whole form, a bala of constituents which reduces toxicity and s effects.

Barberry Root Bark:

Barberry is used to treat general debilities. It also specifically been employed to treat tum of the liver and stomach. In addition, barbe provides a cleansing action through its m laxative effect. As a liver tonic it can prom healthy skin which is only a reflection of body's internal health.

llingia:	Stillingia is an alterative which gradually restores good health. It promotes a healthy liver and treats various skin problems. It is a mild laxative and diuretic further supporting the cleansing action of this formula.
saparilla:	Sarsaparilla root has been used as a blood purifier for centuries. It has been proven to be an excellent treatment for psoriasis, eczema, and other skin disorders. It removes toxins from the body and also serves as an antidote for certain deadly poisons. It protects the liver and improves digestion. As an alterative it gradually restores good health. Sarsaparilla is officially recognized in Britain and Germany.
ckly Ash Bark:	Prickly ash bark is used in Britain to treat various degenerative diseases especially those related with poor circulation. Rheumatism and Raynaud's syndrome are helped as prickly ash improves peripheral circulation. Prickly ash also promotes cleansing by stimulating perspiration. It improves digestion by stimulating saliva and settling the stomach.
scara Sagrada:	Cascara sagrada does not particularly contain direct benefits for degenerative diseases. It does, however, promote cleansing and proper bowel function. Indirectly it helps in conditions of hemorrhoids and ridding the body of gallstones.
rdock Root:	Burdock root is very beneficial in treatment of various skin disorders such as eczema and psoriasis. It is believed to neutralize and eliminate poisons in the body. It has been used in many countries around the world to treat cancers of various types. Its uses in treating degenerative diseases are too numerous to list

here and may not be directly applicable to t
more narrow focus subject of this chapt
Burdock root also improves digestion throu
increasing bile secretion.

Buckthorn Bark:

Buckthorn bark is a member of the same pl:
family as cascara sagrada. Besides buckthor
laxative effect it has been used to tre
inflammatory tumors. It improves digesti
and is believed to be able to remove obstructi
from the liver and gallbladder.

Kelp:

Kelp contains many trace elements that c
assist in the recovery from almost a
degenerative disease. It cleanses the bloodstre:
and improves resistance against disea:
Epidemiological studies demonstrate a stro
link between kelp consumption and reduc
incidence of breast cancer. Kelp can prot
body tissues against radiation exposure. K
contains algin which helps prevent choleste
build-up in the arteries and also binds to tox
and removes them from the body. Algin is v
soothing to the GI tract, which is needed in t
formula since many of the herbs have a mod
laxative effect.

Other Supportive Nutrients

garlic, onion, maitake mushroom, rei:
mushroom, shiitake mushroom, cat's cla
vitamin A, vitamin B-6, vitamin B-12, vitan
C, vitamin D, vitamin E, folic acid, calciu
iodine, magnesium, selenium, zinc, omeg;
and omega 6 fatty acids, acidophil
oligomeric proanthocyanidins, bovine cartila
fruits, vegetables, fiber

30

MENTAL STAMINA

dications:	Poor memory, inability to concentrate, memory loss, amnesia, dementia
commended Formula:	Peppermint leaves, Siberian ginseng, gotu kola, kelp, rosemary leaves, damiana leaves, butternut root bark
sage:	Two to four capsules daily. In more severe cases a person may consume up to 12 capsules daily.
ntraindications:	None
ctor's Review:	Doctors often hear complaints from patients who are experiencing memory loss, poor memory, or an inability to concentrate. Some of these people may also experience other possibly related conditions like poor circulation or tinnitus (ringing in the ear). Memory loss can be caused by many different factors such as head trauma or injury, ischemia or stroke, (a condition where blood flow to parts of the brain has been cut off), poor circulation and oxygen flow to the brain, and organic brain disease. Alcoholism, smoking, and even environmental pollutants may also lead to memory dysfunction. In such cases it is important that the person change environments or habits to stop the progression of the condition. Inability to concentrate may be caused by stress or nervous disorders. This

herbal formula is designed to impro
circulation, and oxygen uptake and transpo
and reduce the effects of stress. This wi
improve the ability to concentrate and reta
memory, and arrest the progression of ag
related memory dysfunctions.

DOCTOR'S NOTES

Peppermint Leaves:

Peppermint improves breathing in two way
First, it opens congested nasal passages allowi
more air to flow into the lungs. The aromat
property in peppermint causes people
breathe more deeply. Second, peppermi
relieves tension and stress which can contribu
to more normal breathing. All this means th
more oxygen will be available for the red bloc
cells to carry throughout the body including
the brain. The anti-stress factor will assist wit
concentration as well. Headaches and migrain
are often the cause of an inability t
concentrate. While the mode of action has y
to be elucidated, peppermint has bee
successful in treating migraines and headache
Peppermint has some general applicatior
which will improve overall health. For exampl
it helps with many disorders such as poc
digestion, heart burn, nausea, and low bil
production and flow. Thus, it is considered t
be a powerful carminative. Improving digestio
will increase the effectiveness of other herbs o
this formula.

Siberian Ginseng:

Siberian ginseng is considered to be a
adaptogen, a substance with the ability t
normalize systems of the body, irrespective o
the direction, deficiency or excess of th
pathologic state. For example, Siberian ginsen

will normalize blood pressure by raising pressure that is too low or reducing pressure that is too high. Clinical studies have demonstrated ginseng's ability to improve physical assertion, mental alertness, and the body's resistance to the effects of stress. It combats physical and especially mental fatigue. Since ginseng reduces serum cholesterol and prevents arteriosclerosis, it can prevent ischemia and stroke. Ginseng will protect the body against the effects of toxic chemicals and radiation, modulate immune system function in fighting disease, and many people claim it slows down the aging process.

Gotu Kola:

Gotu kola is a popular herb used throughout the world but especially in India. Ayurvedic doctors use it as a central nervous system tonic and to improve mental stamina and enhance memory. Clinical studies performed in Europe show gotu kola has the ability to increase circulation. This may prevent senility.

Kelp:

Kelp's high concentration and broad range of trace elements are most likely the reason kelp is considered essential for the nervous system and normal brain function. The algin in kelp soothes and improves GI tract function, and it also binds with cholesterol and toxins to remove them from the body. Kelp improves nutrition and general health.

Rosemary Leaves:

Rosemary helps maintain a healthy nervous system. It assists in combating stress and improves circulation especially in the elderly who may be experiencing chronic poor circulation. Long-term use improves a bad memory. Rosemary contains powerful antioxidants which can reduce damage cause by free radicals. Some claim it relieve headaches.

Damiana Leaves:

Germany's drug regulatory board suggests th use for damiana to include "fortification an stimulation in cases of overwork, mental stres and nervous debility, and for enhancement an maintenance of mental and physical efficiency In Britain it is used as an anti-depressan Damiana prevents constipation and nervou dyspepsia.

Butternut Root Bark:

Butternut root bark has been included in th formula as a laxative to cleanse toxins from th body and to improve health.

Other Supportive Nutrients

ginkgo biloba, bilberry, lady slipper, valeria root, schizandra berry, vitamin B-6, vitamin I 12, vitamin C, vitamin E, folic acid, zin phosphatidyl choline, phosphatidyl serin coenzyme Q10

31

CHOLESTEROL

Indications:	High serum cholesterol, arteriosclerosis.
Recommended Formula:	Apple pectin, hawthorn berries, psyllium husk, devil's claw, juniper berries, ginger root
Dosage:	Two to four capsules daily. Should be used consistently every day.
Contraindications:	None
Doctor's Review:	Cholesterol is often thought of for its negative effects and relation to cardiovascular disease. However, cholesterol is necessary to metabolism and as a precursor in the creation of various important hormones. Cholesterol creates a concern when it becomes too concentrated in the blood. Excessive cholesterol deposition in the arteries is much more likely to occur with elevated blood cholesterol levels. While cholesterol can be taken into the body by consuming animal source foods, it can also be manufactured by the liver and secreted in the bile. This is illustrated by the fact that even when avoiding animal source foods, some people continue to experience elevated serum cholesterol. It is believed that the cause is probably genetic. Although diet plays a significant role in cholesterol regulation, even when excessive amounts are produced in the

liver, avoiding animal source foods has little effect on endogenous cholesterol levels. However, increasing the right type of dietary fiber intake has been shown to make a dramatic difference. This formula contains herbs and plant derivatives found to be exceptionally beneficial in reducing blood cholesterol levels and therefore preventing arteriosclerosis.

DOCTOR'S NOTES

Apple Pectin:

It is well known that fiber plays a vital role in maintaining good health. Fiber maintains a healthy bowel that is much less likely to develop polyps and cancer. Fiber has the ability to intercept cholesterol that has been secreted by the liver in the bile, bond with it and carry it out of the body unabsorbed. Not all types of fiber seem to possess this ability. Those that do are soluble and often able to absorb many times their weight in fluids. Pectin, found in many fruits, is one of those soluble fibers found in many fruits. However, the commonly recognized source is apples. Most people recognize the name pectin from its use as a thickener in many jams and jellies.

Hawthorn Berries:

Hawthorn berry is considered to be the best herbal cardiovascular tonic on the planet. It will treat or prevent many cardiovascular conditions including arteriosclerosis, arrhythmia, weakened heart muscle and angina, high blood pressure and high cholesterol. Hawthorn dilates the coronary vessels improving blood flow and reducing blood pressure and the likelihood of arterial blockage. It will also assist when a heart valve is defective. Hawthorn is highly renowned in Europe for its ability to promote cardiovascular health and is found there in many prescription and over-the-counter medications. Hawthorn should be a part of any formula designed to prevent cardiovascular disease and reduce cholesterol. Hawthorn is also used as a central nervous system tonic and as a mild diuretic.

Psyllium Husk:

Psyllium husk, like pectin, contains a large amount of soluble fiber and, like pectin, carries cholesterol and toxins out of the body. Psyllium is a bulking agent that improves bowel transit time and helps maintain a healthy GI tract.

Devil's Claw:

Devil's claw is an African herb used for various conditions, but is best known for its application with arthritis and inflammation. One of its other uses has been to prevent arteriosclerosis, even though it is not known to have a specific effect on reducing cholesterol. It is also recognized for its ability to clean toxic impurities from the system and has a mild diuretic effect that further supports cleansing.

Juniper Berries:

Juniper berries application in this formula is mainly one of cleansing. Juniper has a strong diuretic effect and is said to improve the kidneys filtration system. Juniper berries have also been used to prevent and treat arteriosclerosis, probably due to the presence of a substance called *beta sitosterol*. Phytosterols (plant sterols) are found throughout the plant kingdom and beta sitosterol is probably the most common phytosterol. These substances are steroid-like compounds found in plants. Beta sitosterol has proven to be very effective in reducing the absorption of dietary cholesterol. The mechanism of action has yet to be defined but is believed to block the cholesterol fro being absorbed or binding the cholesterol achieve the same result.

Ginger Root:

Ginger root is considered to be an activate which helps the other herbs of this formula more effective. It improves circulation digestion, and bowel function.

Other Supportive Nutrients

garlic, ginger, onion, milk thistle, turmeri dandelion, vitamin B-6, vitamin E, folic aci niacin, calcium, chromium, magnesium, zin omega-3 and omega 6 fatty acids, l-carnitin bromelain, glycosaminoglycans, phosphatid choline, phytosterols, beans, brewer's yeas fiber, activated charcoal, soy protein (such tofu)

3 2
HEMORRHOIDS

Indications:	Hemorrhoids, phlebitis (venous inflammation), periodontal inflammations
Recommended Formula:	Witch hazel leaves, mullein leaves, cranesbill, slippery elm bark, plantain, butternut root bark, goldenseal root, peppermint leaves, aloe vera gel
Dosage:	Two to four capsules daily, may be used every day.
Contraindications:	None
Doctor's Review:	Hemorrhoids and phlebitis are conditions of inflamed veins. They can be very painful and create much discomfort. Usually these conditions do not dramatically reduce the quality of life; however, surgical intervention is sometimes required. Many people use stool softeners to reduce the discomfort of hemorrhoids. This formula contains three types of herbs: the astringent herbs that shrink and reduce inflamed veins, herbs that soothe the GI tract and soften stools, and herbs for general function and support.

DOCTOR'S NOTES

Witch Hazel Leaves:	There is probably not an herb that has been employed more often for venous inflammation

than witch hazel. It was listed in the *National Formulary* until 1955 and is still used today in over-the-counter medications to treat hemorrhoids. Witch hazel has a powerful astringent effect which reduces the size of hemorrhoids, and further reduces itching characteristic of hemorrhoids. It also seems to maintain the integrity of the mucosal lining which secretes mucus to help stools leave the body with greater ease. Witch hazel has also been used to treat phlebitis and varicose veins. It promotes wound healing which can prove beneficial in hemorrhoids.

Mullein Leaves:

Mullein leaf contains three to four times the amount of mucilage as other herbs recognized for their mucilage content. Mucilage soothes the GI tract and softens stools. Mullein leaves also contain astringent properties and, like witch hazel, once enjoyed official recognition in the *National Formulary*. Mullein leaf cleanses the body by decreasing bowel transit time and through its mild diuretic property.

Cranesbill:

Cranesbill has gained the respect of herbalists for its powerful astringent properties. It has been used to treat hemorrhoids and periodontal disease characterized by inflammation.

Slippery Elm Bark:

For its benefit with hemorrhoids, the first word in Slippery elm's name is very descriptive. It contains large amounts of mucilage. It helps to heal and restore the GI tract's mucus lining. Slippery elm, like other mucilage containing herbs, soothes and improves the GI tract. It will reduce inflammation and heal sores. This is another herb once listed in the *National Formulary* and still popular today.

antain:

Plantain contains two important healing principles. The first, mucilage, has been sufficiently highlighted in this chapter. The second is *allantoin*. Allantoin has been extensively used to promote wound healing. It is effective internally and externally for ulcers, lacerations, hemorrhoids, periodontal conditions, etc. The *British Herbal Pharmacopeia* recommends plantain and witch hazel be used together to treat hemorrhoids. Plantain's diuretic action also promotes internal health.

ppermint Leaves:

The only direct effect peppermint has on hemorrhoids is as a mild pain reliever. Otherwise peppermint improves digestion by increasing bile production and secretion; reducing gas, belching and flatulence; and settling a spastic colon and stomach. It is considered an activator, increasing the effectiveness of the astringent herbs.

tternut Root Bark:

Butternut root bark is a mild laxative. With the assistance of peppermint, butternut will not cause the painful gripping associated with many laxatives. It softens the stool and relieves pressure from the hemorrhoids. Butternut root bark supports liver function.

ldenseal Root:

Goldenseal root is another astringent herb. It was employed by Russians during World War II to stop the bleeding in wounded soldiers. Goldenseal root strengthens the mucus lining by increasing the cross linking between the various glycoproteins found in the mucus layer. Goldenseal also has a mild laxative effect.

e Vera Gel:

Aloe vera gel is listed last, but is the "icing on the cake." It is extremely soothing and healing to the GI tract. It promotes the growth of th healthy bacterial flora that is so crucial t proper GI tract function. Aloe gel also ca prevent the itching associated with hemorrhoid and has anti-inflammatory properties.

Other Supportive Nutrients

butcher's broom (internal and topical), witc hazel (topical), centella asiatica (topical) vitamin A, vitamin B-complex, vitamin C calcium, bioflavonoids, fiber, fluids

33
ALLERGY

Indications: allergies, hayfever, asthma

Recommended Formula: montmorillonite clay, horehound, mullein leaves, wild cherry bark, barberry root bark, peppermint leaves

Dosage: Four capsules daily. Continue to use as symptoms persist.

Contraindications: None

Doctor's Review: An *allergen* is defined as a substance that causes an allergic response. Allergens can be inhaled from the air as dust, dander, pollen, smoke, perfumes, chemicals, etc. They can come from foods, such as wheat, corn, chocolate, etc., or drugs like penicillin. They can be acquired through infectious organisms such as bacteria, viruses, or parasites. Also, allergens can come from touching things such as plants, animals and chemicals, etc.

Not everyone suffers from allergies. Some people seem to be much more sensitive than others to potential allergens. Some allergies may be genetically passed on. The symptoms of an allergic reaction are often the result of histamine release in the body and usually manifested through respiratory tract in the form of bronchial asthma, hayfever, or allergic rhinitis, etc., and through the skin as eczema hives. Headaches also often accompany allerg response. However, the very best way to avo allergies is to avoid contact with the allerge For some people it may be impossible to avo allergen contact especially if the allergen is the airborne variety, such as polle Nevertheless, when allergens are impossible avoid, there is help. The body usually produc antibodies to combat the allergen. This formu contains herbs and montmorillonite clay th will relieve the symptomatic responses of asthn and nasal congestion, reduce the amount histamine, and improve GI tract health reduce the absorption of allergens into t blood. This formula will also help to reduce t headache quite often associated with allergies.

DOCTOR'S NOTES

Montmorillonite Clay:

Orally consumed montmorillonite clay h great applications for reducing symptoms allergies and the effects of allergens. It absor toxins and reduces histamine. It improves (tract function which will prevent substanc that could cause an allergy response from bei absorbed into the blood. Montmorillonite cl also is an antibacterial which may redu allergic response to toxins produced by bacteri

Horehound:

Horehound has a spasmolytic property whi means that it can reduce spasms. This particularly useful for allergen-induced asthn since asthma is caused when bronchial muscl spasm (contract). Horehound will also redu cough and phlegm produced by the allergen. further cleanses the body of toxins through diuretic properties and ability to produ perspiration. Horehound candy has been popular for years in treating these conditions.

Mullein Leaves:

Mullein, like horehound, has an ability to help control asthma by reducing spasm. This is probably because of its nerve-calming attributes. Mullein leaves are useful in treating bronchitis, sinusitis, and coughs. Many herbalists have found mullein useful in treating headaches and migraines which can result from allergies. Mullein contains high levels of mucilage which can soothe and coat the GI tract and improve bowel function.

Wild Cherry Bark:

Wild cherry bark has been a favorite in cough and cold medicines, but perhaps its greatest contribution in this formula is found in its ability to relax respiratory nerves that cause asthma. Wild cherry bark also improves stomach function and digestion which may be a great help in reducing the allergy response.

Barberry Root Bark:

Barberry root bark's application in this formula is one of general health service. Barberry supports the cleansing of the liver and gall bladder. This will remove toxins and improve digestion. Sometimes improper digestion is the cause of an allergy response. Occasionally, a partly digested protein is absorbed into the blood and since the body doesn't recognize or know how to utilize this partial protein, antibodies are created to remove it. This unwanted protein may be responsible for initiating a histamine response as well. Barberry root bark will stimulate the bowels through its mild laxative properties.

Peppermint Leaves:

Peppermint leaves will make the other herbs of this formula more effective. It has tremendous applications for digestive disorders and disturbances. Anyone who has breathed in its pleasant cooling aroma knows that it has an ability to clear congested nasal passages and improve breathing. Peppermint's volatile oil is described in the *British Herbal Pharmacopeia* as a potent spasmolytic suggesting possible applications with asthma. It has been used to treat headaches.

Other Supportive Nutrients

feverfew leaf, nettle leaf, ginkgo biloba, lobelia, royal jelly, bee pollen, beta carotene, vitamin B-6, vitamin B-12, vitamin E, molybdenum, bioflavonoids, catechin, evening primrose oil, acidophilus, bifidobacteria, combination of quercetin, bromelain, and vitamin C

3 4

HEALING

Indications:	Broken bones, bruises, cuts, wounds, lacerations, ulcers
Recommended Formula:	Horsetail, plantain, slippery elm bark, parsley leaves, marshmallow root, burdock root, myrrh gum
Dosage:	Four to ten capsules daily. Continue to use until healing is complete.
Contraindications:	None
Doctor's Review:	Injuries, whether life-threatening or not, can create hardship or inconvenience. Some injuries will not interfere in any way with lifestyle. Some injuries occur suddenly and others are developed with years of chronic abuse. The latter conditions are usually referred to by a specific disease name, such as cirrhosis of the liver which may be caused by years of alcohol consumption. One-time consumption of alcohol will not cause cirrhosis of the liver, but years of consumption will. Whatever the injury or its source, healing is of prime concern. For those injuries that interfere with lifestyle, the speed of recovery is equally important. This formula contains a mixture of herbs that will assist and accelerate the healing process. It is specifically for broken bones, wounds, abrasions, lacerations, and tissue damaged by inflammation. It can be used when trying to

recover from a disease that includes any of the above conditions.

DOCTOR'S NOTES

Horsetail (Shave Grass):

Horsetail excels in healing various tissues and bones. It contains silica, a mineral found in bones and collagen (connective tissue). Collagen is essentially the structure or glue that holds everything together. Many people believe that bone maintenance and collagen integrity are directly related to the presence of silica. Horsetail has been used extensively to help broken bones heal faster and to stop bleeding. The *British Herbal Pharmacopeia* claims horsetail to be vulnerary, meaning it is healing to fresh cuts or wounds. For wounds subject to possible infections, horsetail mildly increases white blood cell count. Finally horsetail has some diuretic propertie.

Plantain Leaves:

Plantain is also known as "soldier's herb." It got this name from its use in the first aid treatment of wounded soldiers. It is one of the best herbs for healing wounds. Its astringent and hemostatic properties shrink blood vessels and stop bleeding. Plantain leaves contain a substance called *allantoin*. Allantoin is a natural chemical used in the United States and elsewhere to promote wound healing activity. Another great property of plantain is its high mucilage content. Mucilage is a demulcent that is soothing and healing to the GI tract. Is it any wonder why many people have found plantain leaves healing and soothing to peptic ulcers? The mucilage promotes a quicker bowel transit time which further supports the body's cleansing mechanisms.

Slippery Elm Bark: Slippery elm bark contains even higher concentrations of mucilage than plantain discussed in the last paragraph. Most plants containing large amounts of mucilage like plantain, mullein, and slippery elm have been used extensively when applied externally to promote wound healing and reduce inflammation. However, they are just as good for internal use in treating conditions like ulcers, bowel lacerations, and inflammation. Slippery elm has also been used as a convalescent food. The mucilage promotes better bowel function and supports the body's cleansing systems.

Parsley: Parsley is a common garnish used at meal times because parsley freshens the breath, improves stomach function, and reduces foul odors. These same properties make it a great addition to this formula. Parsley will improve GI tract function and help to reduce odors produced by infected wounds. Parsley is full of nutrients that can help in recovery and improving health.

Marshmallow Root: Marshmallow root, like other herbs of this formula, contains large amounts of mucilage. The same benefits described in the preceding paragraphs for mucilage apply to marshmallow root. Marshmallow root has also been employed as a diuretic and to reduce pain and inflammation. Marshmallow is officially recognized for its therapeutic benefits in Belgium, France, Switzerland, Germany, and Britain.

Burdock Root: Burdock root is one of the best herbs to promote healthy skin, general cleansing, and overall health. Burdock root is diaphoretic (promotes perspiration) cleansing toxins from the blood and skin. It also has laxative and diuretic properties stimulating the other two major cleansing systems. It will improve liver function and promote bile secretion. These properties are officially recognized in Belgium, France, Germany, and Britain.

Myrrh Gum:

Myrrh gum has an excellent ability to promote wound healing and is best known for this property. It also exhibits antiseptic and antimicrobial properties. It further fights infections by stimulating production of phagocytes which are cells the body uses to fight infections. Myrrh gum is also soothing and healing to the GI tract helping it to function better.

Other Supportive Nutrients

centella asiatica, turmeric , comfrey (externally applied), vitamin A, vitamin B-1, vitamin C, vitamin E, silica, zinc, pantothenic acid, arginine

35

LOW BLOOD SUGAR

ndications:	Hypoglycemia
ecommended Formula:	Licorice root, gotu kola, Siberian ginseng, ginger root, kelp
osage:	Four to six capsules daily.
ontraindications:	None
octor's Review:	Glucose (blood sugar) is the energy source for the body. The brain cannot function without this vital nutrient. This is why glucose metabolism disorder can be so serious. Hypoglycemia is a glucose metabolism disorder where the pathology is the opposite of diabetes. Diabetes is a condition of too much glucose in the blood because too little insulin is being produced by the pancreas. Hypoglycemia is a condition of too little glucose in the blood often a result of the pancreas producing too much insulin. A diabetic who injects too much insulin can cause a state of hypoglycemia. At one time it was believed that hypoglycemia did not occur except in diabetics who overdosed on insulin.

In non-diabetic individuals hypoglycemia was usually misdiagnosed as other conditions like an anxiety attack. Today, even though more doctors and patients are aware of the possibility |

of hypoglycemia it is often misdiagnosed because symptoms are the same as some other conditions. Fasting or going without food for a few hours can result in inadequate blood sugar which can generate a state of hypoglycemia. Consuming something sweet like orange juice or a candy bar can quickly solve the problem.

Hypoglycemia is potentially a serious condition sometimes resulting in a coma or death. Symptoms of hypoglycemia include extreme fatigue, malaise, weakness, and in more severe cases mental disorders and delirium. This herbal formula provides quick energy by stimulating adrenal glands. It balances blood sugar and improves digestion.

DOCTOR'S NOTES

Licorice Root:

For people in acute hypoglycemic condition licorice root can stimulate adrenal hormone production as a response to provide quick energy. This will allow the person to function until food can be consumed. A hypoglycemic condition can be the result of a dysfunctional digestive system. Poor digestion may not allow the required nutrients to be absorbed and consequently create a condition like that produced by fasting. Licorice root will improve digestion by stimulating the secretion of a soothing mucus in the GI tract. This function is often credited with licorice's clinically proven ability to heal and improve peptic ulcers. People suffering with ulcers may be less likely to eat regularly, possibly creating hypoglycemic conditions. Licorice further stimulates the bowels and kidneys through its laxative and diuretic properties. These actions improve digestion and the elimination of toxin-filled waste. Licorice has an ability to modulate and increase the effectiveness of the other herbs in this formula.

Gotu Kola:

Gotu kola is an herb that sounds suspiciously similar to a popular soft drink. However, gotu kola is not related to that soft drink in any way and certainly does not contain caffeine. Nevertheless, gotu kola has a strong action against mental and physical fatigue. Gotu kola is said to be able to improve energy stores. It has a tonic and an adaptogenic effect on the central nervous system which relies heavily on proper brain function. Gotu kola is a mental stimulant and memory enhancer. Clinical studies in Europe confirm gotu kola's ability to stimulate circulation which may explain many of the above listed benefits. Increased circulation can deliver more nutrients to the various tissues of the body, even when those nutrients are in short supply in the blood. Of course, in a hypoglycemic state, glucose would be in short supply.

Siberian Ginseng:

Siberian ginseng is called an adaptogen which is an innocuous substance that normalizes systems of the body irrespective of the pathology. A common example used to support ginseng's claimed adaptogenic effects is its clinically documented ability to normalize blood sugar levels. Ginseng will bring the blood sugar level to normal whether it is high or low. Ginseng has a similar effect on blood pressure and the central nervous system. Stress and anxiety may have a significant influence on hypoglycemic states since many people are unable to eat when under such conditions. Ginseng has a well

documented ability to fight the effects of stress
Russian athletes have used ginseng not only for
the above properties but also for energy.

Ginger root:

Ginger root's applications in this formula are to
improve digestion and stomach and bowel
function. Ginger will settle nervous stomachs
Ginger improves circulation which will help
make other herbs of this formula more
effective.

Kelp:

Kelp provides many trace elements which are
involved in various metabolic processes. Some
trace elements like chromium are important to
carbohydrate metabolism. Kelp provides a
soothing soluble dietary fiber called *algin*. Algin
improves gastrointestinal function.

Other Supportive Nutrients

artichoke, fritillaria (chuan bei mu), vitamin B
complex, vitamin C, vitamin E, niacinamide
chromium, magnesium, bioflavonoids
methionine, digestive enzymes, acidophilus
fiber

36

MOTION SICKNESS

ndications: Nausea, motion sickness, upset stomach, poor digestion, morning sickness

ecommended Formula: Ginger root, cayenne, licorice root, chamomile

osage: Two to six capsules. May be used every day to prevent or treat nausea. Use maximum dosage if necessary.

ontraindications: None

octor's Review: Most people would admit that there is little worse than being subject to motion sickness and nausea. It's usually not the driver of the car, bus, boat or airplane that experiences nausea, but the passengers. Having motion sickness can be embarrassing since it can come on suddenly and often when other people are near by. Frequently the only relief comes after one turns pale, and then green, and then vomits. This mere description may bring back awful memories. Motion alone is not responsible for all the nausea that people experience. Stomach and digestive disorders, contaminated food, pregnancy, stomach flu, and other conditions have caused their fair share of nausea. Nutritional deficiencies such as a lack of vitamin B-6 may contribute to the condition. Treating the condition can be quite simple, but

preventing it may be a better choice. There
hope in treating the condition using safe a
natural products that have been proven
clinical studies to be more effective th
prescription medications. This formu
contains herbs that have been used f
thousands of years to treat these types
disorders. No automobile glove box
medicine chest should be without it.

DOCTOR'S NOTES

Ginger Root:

The primary herb in this unique formula is t
common household spice ginger. Ginger h
been used on food to flavor and add variety
dishes. The Japanese use it with sushi to fresh
the pallet and improve digestion. In ma
cultures there is no separation between foc
and medicine. In other words, food is t
medicine in treating various conditions. Ging
is definitely a food that when consumed c
have wonderful and powerful influences on t
body. Obviously, its specific applications in tl
formula are similar to its uses in Japan. Ging
is a strong carminative in that it settles to t
stomach. It improves digestion, reduces g
tonifies the intestinal muscle, and stimulates t
liver to bile secretion. The highly acclaimed a
respected British medical journal *Lan*
published a study that found ginger root to
more effective than either dimenhydrate* o
placebo in fighting motion sickness. In anoth
double blind clinical study ginger reduced t
incident of postoperative nausea and vomiti
after major surgery. In another study it reduc
nausea in the most severe cases of morni
sickness, called *hyperemesis gravidarum* whi
can lead to hospitalization and may be fatal

untreated. Enough good things cannot be said about ginger root.

*Dimenhydrinate is sold under the trade name Dramamine and used extensively for motion sickness.

yenne: Cayenne along with licorice and chamomile is used in smaller proportions in this formula compared to ginger root, but it is nevertheless, an important ingredient. Cayenne is not as extensively researched as ginger in the treatment of nausea, but still it seems to have many of the same properties. The British hold cayenne in high regard as it is officially recognized in the *British Herbal Pharmacopeia* as a treatment for colic, flatulence, and poor digestion. It also describes cayenne as a carminative. It will also prevent painful spasms of the stomach and intestines.

orice Root: Licorice root is known as a demulcent which is a substance that soothes the GI tract. It receives this reputation because it stimulates the secretion of mucus in the stomach and bowels. The mucus improves bowel function and protects the stomach and intestines. Licorice has been used by herbalists and natural doctors for years to treat digestive disorders, gastritis, and peptic ulcers. Licorice supports the waste elimination systems of the body through laxative and diuretic actions.

amomile: Chamomile is extremely popular in Germany where it is considered a cure-all. For this formula it imparts a strong carminative action

and relaxes the nerves. Chamomile calm
muscle spasms of the stomach bowels an
throughout the body.

Other Supportive Nutrients

red raspberry leaf, peppermint leaf, fennel seed
angelica, vitamin B-6, magnesium, digestiv
enzymes

37
ANTIOXIDANTS

Indications:	Poor health, pollution, and toxin-exposure aging
Recommended Formula:	Fennel seeds, celery seeds, rosemary extract, cloves, myrrh gum, dandelion root, milk thistle seeds
Dosage:	Four to eight capsules daily. May be used continuously.
Contraindications:	None
Doctor's Review:	There has been a lot of attention given to antioxidants in the media and scientific circles over the past decade. At the root of attention are free radicals. Free radicals are highly reactive and potentially harmful compounds that can cause oxidative damage. Free radicals can be produced in the body as a normal consequence of metabolism. They can also be picked up from air pollutants, alcohol metabolism, cigarette smoke, sunlight, ionizing radiation, and certain medications. Free radicals have been shown to alter DNA strands, destroy cell membranes, and potentially kill cells. No one is completely immune to the effects of free radicals. Everyone is at risk.

Lifestyle factors play a significant role in determining risk to the individual. Poor diet, |

smoking, drinking, and poor environme (occupational and otherwise) can put a pers at greater risk for oxidative damage. Oxidati damage has been implicated in many chron degenerative diseases, including Parkinso disease, cataracts, cancer, emphysem rheumatoid arthritis, and hardening of t arteries.

There is a strong belief that if this harmf oxidation did not occur, people would be bett able to withstand the effects of aging and li much longer. Indeed, some animal studies ha demonstrated a 45 percent increase in longevi brought about by a significant increase antioxidants in the diet.

Nature has provided answers to the problems oxidative damage by supplying substanc called antioxidants in fruits and vegetables ar other plants. The body can produce some of i own antioxidants, and the consumption some plants will help the body produce them larger quantities. Antioxidants are able quench free radicals and render them inacti and harmless. So, do as mom said and consun lots of fruits and vegetables. Intuitively sl knew what she was talking about.

Some of the most powerful antioxidants foods are found in spices. Before the inventic of the ice box, herbs and spices were used preserve foods from microbial contaminatic and rancidification (oxidation). Herbs an spices have been used by many cultures prepare and preserve bodies after death. Th more recognized antioxidants in plants includ vitamin C, vitamin E, and carotenes. Howeve so many antioxidants are found in the pla kingdom that even with today's technology and resources it would be an impossible task to find and identify all of them. Many plants and antioxidants are found to be hundreds of times more powerful than the above mentioned vitamin antioxidants. This herbal formula is designed to supply powerful antioxidant activity to quench free radicals and prevent the consequential damage. This is accomplished by relying on spices known to possess powerful antioxidants. Most experts suggest that eating a healthy diet should be the first line of defense. This formula can contribute to and become a part of a healthy diet and may be used to support any of the herbal formulas described in this book.

DOCTOR'S NOTES

Fennel Seeds:

Plant seeds have been known to contain antioxidant compounds and activity. Plant seeds contain these antioxidants as a means of self-preservation. Vitamin E is often found in the oil fraction of this seed. Fennel seeds also contain antioxidant vitamins and other more powerful antioxidant compounds like the flavonoids, quercetin kaempferol, and isorhamnetin.

Celery Seeds:

Celery seeds contain powerful antioxidants and have been used for hundreds and possibly thousands of years in the preservation of foods. Patents were granted in the late 1930s for antioxidant activity made up of a combination of celery, sage, and cloves. Indoles are compounds found in many plants, spices, and vegetables including celery. Indoles can prevent the destructive nature of toxins and carcinogens.

Rosemary:

Rosemary is found to contain very powerf
antioxidants. In fact, rosemary's antioxida
effect has been shown to be more powerful th:
that of BHT (Butylated Hydroxy-toulene)
vitro. About 10 percent of the dry rosema
leaves are antioxidants.

Cloves:

Cloves also contain strong antioxidants. Clo
derivatives were part of the antioxidant formu
that was patented in the late 1930s. Clov
impart a strong carminative action on t
stomach.

Myrrh Gum:

Myrrh has been used since ancient times as :
ingredient in perfumes and incense. It was a
extensively employed in the barrier process
an embalming preservative. Today it is used f
various ailments and also for its antioxida
properties.

Dandelion Root:

Dandelion root is used in this formula in
supporting role. It cleanses and strengthens t
liver and digestive function. It will also clean
the bowels and blood with its laxative a
diuretic properties.

Milk Thistle Seed:

Milk thistle seeds are best known for the
ability to improve liver health and functio
Milk thistle contains antioxidants, but mi
thistle excels at increasing the liver's ability
produce glutathione peroxidase one of t
body's most powerful antioxidants.

Other Supportive Nutrients

bilberry, carotene, vitamin E, vitamin C, niaci
chromium, selenium, bioflavonoids,
glutathione, l-cysteine, alpha-lipoic acid, gre
tea extract, oligomeric proanthocyanidins

3 8
HAIR

dications:

Dry, brittle or dull hair, hair loss, male pattern baldness, thinning hair

commended Formula:

Saw palmetto berries, horsetail (shave grass), watercress, juniper berries, white willow bark, rosemary leaves, burdock root, mullein leaves

osage:

Four to eight capsules daily. Should be used every day. A lower dosage may be used when desired results have been achieved.

ontraindications:

None

octor's Review:

Hair loss is a great concern to many people. The rate of hair loss varies from person to person. Male pattern baldness is a condition where a person may have ample facial and body hair, but experiences hair loss on the scalp. It is caused by the DHT (Dihydro-testosterone) hormone's reaction with the hair follicle. Even though the condition is called Male Pattern Baldness, women with elevated levels of DHT may also experience the same condition but usually to a lesser extent. Women who experience male pattern baldness often have more facial hair than other women. DHT is produced when the lesser active testosterone is acted upon by an enzyme called *5-alpha reductase*. DHT will bond to a site on the follicle and cause the follicle to slowly die. On⦁ the follicle is dead, the hair is permanently lost

There are various other forms of hair lo besides male pattern baldness. Hair loss may ⅼ caused by hormonal changes and disorde (such as those that occur after a woman h given birth), serious illness, drugs, genet factors, radiation, and the aging process itself.

A person may experience hair problems witho⦁ hair loss. Dry, dull, brittle hair can indica⦁ among other things poor nutrition. Goc nutrition is vital for healthy hair. This formu contains herbs that can improve digestion ar liver function which have a strong impact c nutrition and hair health. This formula w⦁ provide nutrients needed for healthy hair, and will balance the body's hormones.

DOCTOR'S NOTES

Saw Palmetto Berries:

Saw palmetto berries have historically been use to treat urinary tract disorders in men an women. This use has undergone scientif scrutiny particularly in Europe. Today, sa palmetto is used to treat enlarged prosta⦁ conditions in men and dysmenorrhea an pelvic congestion in women. Scientific studi have demonstrated that saw palmetto berri⦁ work partly by inhibiting 5-alpha-reductas⦁ This means that less testosterone will ⅼ converted to DHT. Less DHT can mean le⦁ hair loss in men and women prone to ma⦁ pattern baldness. It may also mean less faci⦁ hair for women. Saw palmetto berries seem ⦁ exert a hormone balancing effect irrespective ⦁ gender.

Horsetail (Shave Grass): Folklore suggests horsetail has been used by herbalists and natural doctors to strengthen hair, reduce split ends, and hair loss. Horsetail contains large amounts of silica which is believed to be an important nutrient for hair, nails, skin, and bones which may explain horsetail folklore. Horsetail will help clean toxins from the body by stimulating urine flow.

Watercress: Watercress is used to improve digestion. It also contains a rich source of nutrients which can improve overall health and support the hair.

Juniper Berries: Hair loss can be caused by malnutrition which can be caused by digestive disorders. Juniper berries have an ability to improve digestion in the absence of sufficient hydrochloric acid. Hydrochloric acid is primarily used to break down proteins. Poor protein digestion can have a dramatic impact on hair health. Juniper berry is best known as a diuretic, and it can cause an increase in the rate of kidney filtration. Cleansing will improve overall health.

White Willow Bark: White willow bark is best known as a natural pain reliever. However, it has also been used to promote a healthy scalp and prevent dandruff and eczema.

Rosemary Leaves: Rosemary leaves improve digestion by stimulating bile flow and settling the stomach. Rosemary has been used as a hair tonic to prevent baldness. Rosemary leaves contain powerful antioxidants which can reduce the effects of aging and possibly reduce age-related hair loss.

Burdock Root:

Burdock root plays a supportive role in th formula by cleansing the internal bod' Burdock root mildly increases bowel ai kidney action. It also reduces the load on t liver by stimulating perspiration.

Mullein Leaves:

Mullein leaves, like burdock root, suppo internal health. Mullein leaves are exceptiona¹ high in mucilage. Mucilage is a demulcent that it is soothing to the GI tract and thus supports proper GI tract function. It has a mi laxative effect.

Other Supportive Nutrients

Pygeum africanum, vitamin A, vitamin complex, vitamin C, copper, iodine, iro· magnesium, manganese, silica, sulfur, zin· omega 6 fatty acids, l-cysteine, protein

39

DEPRESSION

Indications: Depression, anxiety, chronic fatigue syndrome, mononucleosis, thoughts of worthlessness or suicide

Recommended Formula: St. John's wort, kava, Siberian ginseng, gotu kola, kelp, ginger root, butternut root bark

Dosage: Four to eight capsules daily

Contraindications: None

Doctor's Review: Depression seems to be more prevalent today than it was years ago and affects people of all ages. Obviously depression is a problem for the sufferer, but it can also be a problem for others who are associated with the sufferer. The intensity of depression can vary from mild to extremely severe where it can lead to serious problems including suicide. Causes of depression are also varied and include chemical imbalances, medications, stress, and mental disorders.

Fortunately, there are several excellent herbs that are very beneficial in treating depression. This formula can increase sense of well-being and happy contentment, improve mental function and stamina, and provide energy. It will also cleanse toxins from the body that may be contributing to the depression.

DOCTOR'S NOTES

St. John's Wort:

Perhaps St. John's wort is the best herb fo
treating depression. It is widely used in Europ
for treating mild to moderate depression. Th
official German monograph indicates St. John'
wort's applications include depressive states
fear, and nervous disturbances.

Another noteworthy property of St. John's wor
is its ability to fight viral infections. People wh
suffer from viral conditions such as chroni
fatigue syndrome, mononucleosis, herpe
simplex, and AIDS are often depressed. In thes
conditions, St. John's wort will provide moo
elevation while it fights the virus.

Kava:

Kava is used by people throughout the Soutl
Pacific where it is an important ceremonia
drink. People who consume kava note a sense o
well-being and happy contentment. After mucl
clinical research, several European countrie
approved kava for the treatment of nervou
anxiety and restlessness.

It was noted in some of the clinical studies tha
symptoms associated with anxiety—hear
palpitation, headaches, and dizziness—wer
greatly reduced by kava. Other studies indicate
mood improvements. Its active principles ar
called *kavalactones.*

Siberian Ginseng:

Siberian ginseng will help combat depression i
three ways. First, Siberian ginseng has
clinically supported reputation as a stres
fighter. It helps the body cope with stress an
maintain proper function when subjected t
stressful environments. Second, Siberia

ginseng is known for its ability to energize the body and increase stamina. Third, it strengthens mental function and reduces mental fatigue. Disorders such as neurosis and hyperchondriasis are helped by Siberian ginseng.

otu Kola:

Ayurvedic doctors use gotu kola as a central nervous system tonic, to improve mental stamina, and enhance memory. Gotu kola, through clinical studies, has been shown to improve circulation. This, combined with its diuretic effect, makes gotu kola an efficient cleanser of toxins from the body that otherwise may contribute to depression.

elp:

Kelp provides organic iodine which promotes healthy thyroid function. A dysfunctional thyroid has been associated with depression, lethargy, and general malaise. Kelp further provides trace elements that may be lacking in the diet. Thus, kelp may help to provide chemical balance to the body. Kelp also contains algin which improves the function of and soothes the gastrointestinal tract. Kelp's diuretic property further contributes to the cleansing action of this formula.

inger Root:

Ginger root stimulates digestion and circulation. These properties increase the effectiveness of the other herbs in this formula. Some herbalists have also suggested that ginger root helps to fight depression.

utternut Root Bark:

Butternut root bark is a mild laxative and, therefore, supports the body's cleansing systems. This laxative effect is so gentle that it may go unnoticed by the user.

Other Supportive Nutrients

ginkgo biloba, lady slipper, vitamin B-
vitamin B-2, vitamin B-6, vitamin B-12, fo
acid, calcium, iron, magnesium, omega 6 fat
acids, dl-phenylalanine, d-phenylalanine,
tyrosine

40

IMMUNE DEFICIENCY

Indications:

Weak constitution, immune deficiency, chronic disease, AIDS

Recommended Formula:

Astragalus, Siberian ginseng, shiitake mushroom, reishi mushroom, St. John's wort, schizandra, ginger root, licorice root, Irish moss

Dosage:

Four to eight capsules daily. For chronic conditions, use every day for several months.

Contraindications:

None

Doctor's Review:

Since the discovery of AIDS, many Americans have become more aware of the importance of the body's immune system. AIDS has painfully taught the difficult lesson that life can be short without proper immune function. Immune deficiency is a significantly threatening problem whenever disease is allowed to progress.

Of course, many people have suppressed immune function for various reasons unrelated to HIV. Generally, the degree of suppression influences the degree of disease. Some people are unable to get the upper hand on sickness, experiencing one ailment after another. Commonly, this type of immune deficient condition is referred to as a weak or frail constitution.

The body's defense mechanism is complex. In some cases an organism or virus must penetrate several lines of defense in order to cause a problem. Some defense lines are learned such as washing hands to prevent the spread of disease-causing germs and properly storing and preparing food to prevent food-borne illness. However, the body has many built-in defense systems which, when functioning properly, can lead to a long, healthy life.

The body's defenses include the skin, mucus layers covering infection-susceptible tissues, white blood cells (leukocytes), and interferon. Leukocytes are divided into two classes called *granulocytes* and *agranulocytes*. These two classes are further divided into smaller groups.

Granulocytes are primarily *phagocytic* which mean they have the ability to ingest particulate substances. Leukocytes with this ability are often called *phagocytes* and their action *phagocytosis*. Granulocytes include *juvenile neutrophils, segmented neutrophils, basophils,* and *eosinophils.* Each of these performs a specific task. Neutrophils neutralize bacteria and small particles by ingesting them. Basophils are believed to deliver anticoagulants to facilitate blood clot absorption. Eosinophils increase in numbers with asthma and certain infections. Even though their action is not well understood, they probably keep these conditions under control.

The agranulocytes include *monocytes* and large and small *lymphocytes.* Monocytes are able to ingest large particles such as foreign proteins and peptides while lymphocytes produce antibodies and are important to cellular immunity .

Interferon is a protein or proteins formed when cells are exposed to viruses. Noninfected cells will become immune to the virus when exposed to interferon. Interferon interferes with the virus's ability to perpetuate.

If the body's ability to properly produce interferon or a class or subclass of leukocyte is impaired, the health of the body may be successfully challenged by intruding disease. Therefore, it is easy to understand the critical nature of healthy immune function.

Botanicals have been employed by many cultures to support and improve immune function. This formula contains some of the best herbs known to build and strengthen the body's resistance to disease. It is ideal for sufferers of chronic immune deficiency and may be used daily.

DOCTOR'S NOTES

Astragalus:

Astragalus is one of the most popular herbs in Chinese medicine where it is regarded as a tonic, energizer, and potent immune builder. Recent scientific studies have confirmed astragalus benefit for immune function. Astragalus has been shown to increase phagocytosis and interferon production. In another study it was shown to increase the action of interleukin II, a cancer chemotherapeutic agent. Astragalus has also been shown to increase T-lymphocytes of the helper type. These lymphocytes are responsible for activating immune response. The compounds believed responsible for astragalus's activity are high molecular weight polysaccharides. Astragalus also has a diuretic effect which will assist in cleansing the internal body.

Siberian Ginseng:	Chronic stress can lead to illness by eroding immune function. Siberian ginseng has a clinically supported reputation as a stress fighter. It will also improve energy levels, and mental function and stamina which are often lacking in chronically ill people. Siberian ginseng has a history of use in successfully treating various diseases including certain types of cancer. In the past ten years, research has demonstrated Siberian ginseng's ability to increase important T-lymphocytes of the helper variety. These lymphocytes are significantly reduced in HIV infections.
Shiitake Mushroom:	During the Ming dynasty in China the noted herbalist Wu Ming referred to shiitake mushrooms as the "elixir of life." Shiitake mushrooms have received considerable attention for their immune system building effects. This mushroom has been scientifically studied and shown to stimulate interferon production and increase helper T-lymphocytes. Shiitake is very safe and is used in foods around the world.
Reishi Mushroom:	Reishi mushroom has similar applications to shiitake mushroom. It has been called the "mushroom of immortality." While this statement certainly exaggerates the mushroom's capabilities, it demonstrates the high regard that people have for it.
St. John's Wort:	St. John's wort contributes to this formula in two ways. First, St. John's has potent antiviral activity. It has been used to fight the viruses associated with chronic fatigue, herpes simplex, mononucleosis, and AIDS. Second, St. John's wort has clinically proven antidepressive activity which may be of benefit to the chronically ill.

Ginger Root:

Ginger root has a strong carminative (settling to gastrointestinal tract) action. It is also one of the best herbs for stimulating and improving digestion and circulation. These properties will improve the effectiveness of the other herbs in this formula. And for those people who experience nausea with their chronic ailments, ginger root has been clinically proven more effective than prescription medication for nausea.

Licorice Root:

Licorice root is one of the most used plants in Chinese medicine and is referred to as the "Great Adjunct." One reason is because it increases the effectiveness of other herbs. However, animal studies have shown licorice to enhance the production of interferon and macrophage (a large phagocyte) activity. It inhibits herpes type viruses and effectively treats cold sores. Licorice has a demulcent property soothing to the gastrointestinal tract. It is also a mild laxative which will support toxin removal from the body.

Irish Moss:

Irish moss contains iodine and large amounts of mucilage. A deficiency in iodine has been associated with reduction in the ability of some leukocytes to fight bacterial infections. Mucilage is nutritious and soothing to the gastrointestinal tract.

Other Supportive Nutrients

garlic, maitake mushroom, pau d'arco, cat's claw, elderberry, sarsaparilla, vitamin A, beta carotene, vitamin B-complex, vitamin C, vitamin D, vitamin E, copper, iodine, iron, magnesium, selenium, zinc, dimethylglycine, omega-6 fatty acids, l-carnitine, taurine, n-acetyl cysteine, acidophilus

Glossary of Terms

Adaptogen: an agent that increases resistance to stress and that can help restore homeostasis to a person independent of the direction of abnormality.

Alterative: an agent that cleanses the body and stimulates the efficient removal of waste products, and that helps restore the body to a normal or homeopathic state.

Anecdotal: relating or pertaining to biographical stories or incidents.

Aphrodisiac: an agent that stimulates sexual desire.

Aromatic: an agent that contains volatile, essential oils which aids digestion and relieves gas.

Astringent: an agent that has a constricting or binding effect, such as one that checks hemorrhages or secretions by coagulating proteins.

Benign: a bitter secretion of the liver which aids the body in the metabolism of fats.

Bile: a bitter secretion of the liver which aids the body in the metabolism of fats.

Capillary: a tiny blood vessel which joins arteries and veins.

Carminative: an agent that relieves intestinal gas pain and distension.

Cholagogue: an agent that stimulates bile flow from the gallbladder and bile ducts into the duodenum.

Collagen: a fibrous protein that is the main constituent of connective tissue such as tendons and ligaments.

Demulcent: an agent that softens and soothes damaged or inflamed surfaces, such as the mucous membranes that line the gastrointestinal tract.

Diaphoretic: an agent that causes perspiration and increases elimination through the skin.

Diuretic: an agent that increases the secretion and flow of urine.

Electrolyte: an element or compound that is able, when dissolved in a liquid, to conduct an electric current in the body.

Emollient: an agent that softens and soothes inflamed tissue; it also softens and protects the skin.

Endogenous: originating from within the body; such as a disease caused by the failure of an organ or system.

Epidemiological studies: studies concerning the incidence, prevalence, spread, prevention and control of disease in a community or specific group of individuals.

Exogenous: originating outside the body, such as a disease produced from external causes, as from a virus or bacterium.

Expectorant: an agent that encourages the loosening and removal of mucous from the respiratory tract.

Gastrointestinal: pertaining to the digestive and eliminating systems of the body , which extends from the mouth all the way to the anus.

Glycoprotein: a carbohydrate bound to a protein which is found in the mucous membranes of the body. Its function is to lubricate areas such as the joints and intestinal tract.

Hemostatic: an agent that stops bleeding.

Histamine: a compound produced in the body by the breakdown of histidine which contributes to allergic reactions.

Intestinal flora: microorganisms which inhabit the intestines and contribute to the body's natural immunity.

Malaise: a feeling of physical weakness or general discomfort, which often heralds the onset of an illness.

Mucilage: complex sugar molecules that are soft and slippery and protect mucous membranes and inflamed tissues.

Pharmacopoeia: a publication which describes strengths, standards of purity, descriptions, etc. of plants or drugs.

Platelet aggregation: when blood platelets group together, causing coagulation of the blood.

Prophylaxis: contributing to the prevention of infection and disease.

Psychogenic: a disease or anything that originates within the mind.

Putrefaction: decomposition of organic matter, especially by proteins, by the action of bacteria. This results in foul-smelling compounds.

Spasmolytic: having the ability to relieve spasms.

Tonic: a substance that exerts a gentle strengthening effect on the body.

Trace elements: elements essential for health, but which are needed in only very small amounts.

Index

References

Bradley, Peter R., ed. *British Herbal Compendium.* Vol. 1, British Herbal Medicine Association. London.

British Herbal Pharmacopoeia. British Herbal Medicine Association. London.

Duke, James A., Ph.D. *CRC Handbook of Medicinal Herbs.* CRC Press. Boca Raton, Florida.

Hutchens, Alma R. *Indian Herbalogy of North America.* Merco. Windsor, Ontario, Canada.

Kloss, Jethro. *Back to Eden.* Back to Eden Books. Loma Linda, California.

Lust, John B., N.D., D.B.M. *The Herb Book.* Bantam Books. New York.

Meyer, Joseph E. *The Herbalist.* Meyerbooks. Glenwood, Illinois

Mowrey, Daniel B., Ph.D. *The Scientific Validation of Herbal Medicine.* Keats Publishing. New Canaan, Connecticut.

Pearson, Durk, and Sandy Shaw. *Life Extension.* Warner Books. New York.

Pizzorno, Joseph E. Jr., N.D. *A Textbook of Natural Medicine.* Vol. 1–2, John Bastyr College Publications. Seattle Washington.

Tyler, Varro E., Ph.D. *The New Honest Herbal.* George F. Stickley Co. Philadelphia, Pennsylvania.

Werbach, Melvyn R., M.D. *Nutritional Influences on Illness.* Third Line Press. Tarzana, California.